THE ENABLING ENVIRONMENT FOR DISASTER RISK FINANCING IN THE KYRGYZ REPUBLIC

COUNTRY DIAGNOSTICS ASSESSMENT

FEBRUARY 2025

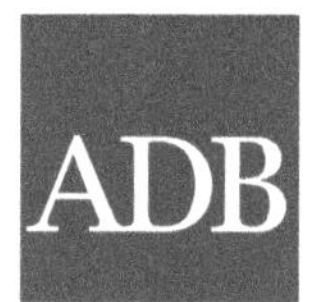

ASIAN DEVELOPMENT BANK

Contents

Tables, Figures, and Boxes

Acknowledgments

This report was prepared under the Technical Assistance (TA)-6561 REG: Strengthening the Enabling Environment for Disaster Risk Financing (Phase 2). The TA was executed by the Asian Development Bank (ADB) in collaboration with the Government of the Kyrgyz Republic.

Charlotte Benson, principal disaster risk management specialist, Climate Change and Disaster Risk Management Division, Climate Change and Sustainable Development Department, ADB and Arup Chatterjee, principal financial sector specialist, Finance Sector Office, Sectors Group, ADB, oversight provided direction and technical advice for this report.

The document benefited significantly from discussions with and comments from Kanopan Lao-Araya, Country Director, ADB Kyrgyz Republic Resident Mission (KYRM), Central and West Asia Department (CWRD); Gulkayr Tentieva, Senior Economic Officer, KYRM; Bobir Gafurov, Public Management Specialist, Public Management, Financial Sector, and Trade Division (CWPF), CWRD; Yasmin Saddiqi, Director, Environment, Natural Resources and Agriculture Division (CWER), CWRD; Nathan Rive, Senior Climate Change Specialist, CWER, CWRD; Kathleen Anne Coballes, Climate Change Officer, CWER, CWRD; and Brian Chin, Senior Health Specialist, Social Sector Division (CWSS), CWRD.

The report was produced by a team of ADB consultants comprising international consultants Rodolfo Wehrhahn (team leader, insurance and capital market regulatory specialist), Roman Shynkarenko (agriculture insurance specialist), Hamid Rohilai (public finance management specialist), and Christian Pfleiderer (health insurance specialist); national consultant Bakhtyiar Bakasuulu (insurance industry specialist); and ADB consultant Maria Cristina Pascual (project coordinator).

The report benefited extensively from productive interactions with a number of representatives from key organizations to whom the team would like to express great appreciation for the time dedicated and the candidness of their opinions.

Government Agencies
Ministry of Finance
Ministry of Economy and Commerce
Chamber of Accounts of the Kyrgyz Republic
Ministry of Labor, Social Security and Migration
Ministry of Emergency Situation
Ministry of Health
Ministry of Agriculture
Ministry of Transport and Communications
Agency for Hydrometeorology
State Service for Regulation and Supervision of the Finance Market

Mandatory Health Insurance Fund
Social Fund of the Kyrgyz Republic
State Insurance Organization

Private Sector
Association of Legal Entities of Insurance Companies
Aga Khan Foundation
Au Garant
ATN Polis
Salym Finance
Oxus Kyrgyz
Jubilee Kyrgyzstan Insurance Company

Development Partners
United Nations Children's Fund
UN World Food Programme

Abbreviations

ADB	–	Asian Development Bank
AYII	–	area yield index insurance
CAREC	–	Central Asia Regional Economic Cooperation
CDC	–	Center for Disease Control and Prevention
COVID-19	–	coronavirus disease
DRF	–	disaster risk financing
FSA	–	Financial Service Authority
FSAP	–	Financial Sector Assessment Program
GDP	–	gross domestic product
IAIS	–	International Association of Insurance Supervisors
GIZ	–	German Agency for International Cooperation
ICP	–	Insurance Core Principles
IFC	–	International Finance Corporation
IFRS	–	International Financial Reporting Standards
IMF	–	International Monetary Fund
IPSAS	–	International Public Sector Accounting Standards
KSE	–	Kyrgyz Stock Exchange
NBFSA	–	Non-Bank Financial Services Authority
ODA	–	official development assistance
PA	–	personal accident
R&D	–	research and development
RBC	–	risk-based capital framework
SOEs	–	state-owned enterprises
SSS	–	Social Security System
TA	–	technical assistance
VAT	–	value-added tax
WHO	–	World Health Organization

Currency Equivalent

Currency unit = som

$1	=	Som95.47
Som1	=	$0.0104739

Executive Summary

The Kyrgyz Republic is among the most disaster-prone countries in the world due to natural hazards that include earthquakes, floods, landslides, mudslides, avalanches, snowstorms, mountain lake spills, droughts, and epidemics. It experiences disasters every year that result in significant financial losses. The coronavirus disease (COVID-19) pandemic has had a long-lasting and severe impact on the economy through medical costs, lockdowns that reduced productivity and created unemployment, and trade and supply chain interruptions. Each of these has put the country's financing capacity to the test.

This country diagnostics assessment focuses on disaster risk financing (DRF) and how it is used in the Kyrgyz Republic. It examines whether it is making efficient and effective use of existing financing instruments and introducing new ones to enhance financial resilience to disasters, epidemics, and pandemics. The assessment covers risk retention and risk transfer instruments to the insurance, reinsurance, and capital markets.

An Asian Development Bank–World Bank methodology is applied to assess possible impediments to the effective functioning of self-insurance or risk retention financing instruments of the government. This methodology has been adapted to include pandemic and epidemic risk. The disaster risk retention instrument insights gained from the questionnaire responses are complemented by analyzing existing publicly available information, carrying out discussions with national and local government agencies, as well as exploring international best practice.

The modified version of the W&W Development Framework is used to accommodate international good practice and public and private sector stakeholders' inputs. This allows insight into existing or perceived demand and supply barriers restricting the development of an enabling environment for disaster risk transfer instruments. Six areas relevant for developing insurance and capital market solutions for DRF are reviewed within this framework. These include government policy; social protection policy; unlicensed competition; economic conditions; credibility of the insurance, reinsurance, and capital markets providers; and product appeal.

A risk layered structure is proposed to stimulate, develop, and implement financially sustainable and scalable DRF strategies and solutions. The assessment makes recommendations to enhance the enabling environment for public sector DRF instruments, insurance, reinsurance, and capital markets solutions. Key recommendations are as follows:

Key Recommendations to Stregthen the Enabling Environment for Disaster Risk Financing

Issues/Recommendations	Timing[a] and References
Existing budget allocations are insufficient to enable the government to retain fiscal shocks arising from annual disaster events.	Immediate. Para. 51
Explore options for securing a contingent disaster financing facility.	
The financing of infrequent but severe disaster events needs attention.	Near term. Para. 52
Acquire risk transfer solutions for extreme but infrequent disaster events.	
There is limited information related to fiscal risks arising from disasters.	Near term. Para. 53
Enhance the collection of information and related analysis regarding fiscal risks arising from disaster.	
Investments in weather monitoring infrastructure are insufficient.	Near term. Para. 67
Increase investments in weather monitoring infrastructure to support disaster risk financing (DRF) mechanisms.	
Availability and access to disaster risk models provides the basis for a robust DRF strategy and the pricing of insurance premiums.	Medium term. Para. 69
Collect necessary data from relevant government ministries on disaster events affecting the country.	
Develop an open source disaster risk model covering all major hazards including pandemics and/or epidemics faced by the country.	
The existing health information landscape and pandemic surveillance data systems are still fragmented and partly manually operated.	Near term. Para. 70
Develop and implement a health information systems integration strategy.	
The agriculture sector is affected by natural hazards—expected to occur more frequently and severely due to climate change—requiring special attention to enhance data availability.	Immediate. Para. 71–72
Support the development of databases for agriculture risk management and increase the capacity of the Hydrometeorological Service.	
The lack of disaster risk insurance of public assets, including the large number of state-owned enterprises, leaves the government exposed to possible severe losses.	Near term. Para. 82
Using the risk layered approach, evaluate the use of insurance for critical public assets as a starting point to securing insurance cover.	

continued on next page

Table *continued*

Issues/Recommendations	Timing[a] and References
The Compulsory Disaster Property Law and its implementation show deficiencies in achieving its objective for providing universal property insurance.	Immediate. Para. 83–84
Increase the resilience of the State Insurance Organization.	
Improve State Insurance Organization processes to increase efficiency and acceptability.	
Enforce the law to improve its outreach.	
Enhance the Compulsory Disaster Property Law benefits to target different sectors of the population.	
Systems for pandemic preparedness are in place, but implementation is weak.	Near term. Para. 91
Improve the integration of existing health emergency pillars.	
The total cost of the country's health response to coronavirus disease (COVID-19) is unclear, which makes understanding future epidemic and pandemic disaster-risk funding needs challenging.	Near term. Para. 93
Develop pandemic and/or epidemic financing plan based on the risk-layered framework.	
Increasing the financial protection for farmers is critical.	Near term. Para. 111
Develop the DRF framework for agriculture based on the risk-layered approach.	
The significant amount of work of the Financial Service Authority to regulate, supervise, and develop the insurance sector in a sound manner requires important capacity building and significant resources.	Immediate. Para. 117
Assess the current and future resources and expertise needed for an effective supervision.	
The size of the insurance sector limits its importance in terms of disaster risk financial protection.	Immediate. Para. 123
Develop a strategy to grow the insurance sector and implement it.	
The development of agriculture insurance as a globally proven DRF tool is critical to support sustainable farming.	Near term. Para. 126
Develop agriculture insurance including crop, livestock, and fishery.	
While the use of pools is common practice in several countries to deal with insurance market failures in areas like agriculture, energy, aviation, or disasters, the Kyrgyz Republic does not use this type of instrument.	Near term. Para. 130
Consider the setting up of effective risk pools to support the development of agriculture insurance and disaster risks products.	

continued on next page

Table   *continued*

Issues/Recommendations	Timing[a] and References
The development of agriculture insurance products faces serious challenges requiring several actions to be taken.	Near term. Para. 134
Develop a suite of standard insurance products for the agriculture insurance program.	
Gradually introduce the products, starting from the larger crop and livestock types.	
Develop standard underwriting, especially standard loss adjustment procedures for agriculture insurance.	

[a] "Immediate" is within 1 year, "near term" is 1–3 years.
Source: Asian Development Bank.

Introduction

1.1 Background

1.   **Disasters triggered by natural hazards, epidemics, and pandemics delay long-term development and hamper efforts to reduce poverty in developing countries in Asia and the Pacific.** Disasters set back development, directly damaging and destroying infrastructure and disrupting related economic activities and the provision of services. They place countries on lower long-term growth trajectories, push vulnerable communities deeper into poverty, and force adjustments in short- and longer-term development targets and goals. They can place significant fiscal strain on governments, businesses, and individual households, particularly if financial preparedness arrangements are limited. Delays and shortages in funding can also significantly exacerbate the consequences of direct physical losses, extending the time to rebuild. Government officials, policymakers, and insurance regulators from developing countries across Asia and the Pacific are therefore seeking to strengthen their financial preparedness for disasters, epidemics, and pandemics, smoothing the cost of events over time and ensuring timely availability of post-disaster funding. A strong enabling environment for such financing, including for stimulation of commercial risk transfer markets, is a priority prerequisite for achieving this. This report refers to such funding as disaster risk financing (DRF).

2.   **The severity and long-lasting duration of the coronavirus disease (COVID-19) pandemic severely tested the financial resilience of countries across the globe.** Box 1 highlights the economic impacts of the pandemic and the unprecedented financing challenges it created in addressing health needs, providing livelihoods and business relief support, and maintaining economic stability.

Box 1: The Global Impact of the COVID-19 Pandemic

The sheer scale of the interventions needed to confront the health and economic consequences of the coronavirus disease (COVID-19) pandemic challenged the capacity to manage resources effectively and equitably in unprecedented ways. By the end of 2020, governments had already mobilized $14 trillion in fiscal policy responses of different types. These included additional spending measures, tax relief programs, loans and loan guarantees—all to fund health services, address income losses, and keep economies afloat. Fiscal responses differed across countries—and were much larger in richer countries—but everywhere they have represented a very significant departure from normal fiscal policy processes.[a]

continued on next page

Box   *continued*

The COVID-19 pandemic is the most devastating shock to hit the global economy since the Second World War. Policies to contain the virus deeply undercut economic activity. The recession's unique character posed unfamiliar policy challenges. On the demand side, lockdowns and social distancing measures triggered a sudden stop in spending and made it highly insensitive to policy stimulus. On the supply side, containment measures directly hindered production, with the repercussions spreading through local and global supply chains. The overall damage could still leave permanent scars if persistent unemployment and bankruptcies follow.[b]

Across Asia and the Pacific, COVID-19 hit poor and vulnerable hard, particularly informal workers. Estimates suggest that in the second quarter 2020 working hours dropped 13.5% in the region, equivalent to 235 million full-time jobs.[c]

This dislocation exposed massive protection gaps in business continuity risk. Less than 1% of the estimated $4.5 trillion global pandemic-induced gross domestic product loss for 2020 is likely to be covered, reflecting pre-COVID-19 coverage exclusions and restrictions and the niche character of business interruption insurance, which accounts for less than 2% of the world's property and casualty insurance market.[d]

Sources:
[a] International Budget Partnership. 2021. Managing Covid Funds: The Accountability Gap. https://internationalbudget.org/covid/wp-content/uploads/2021/05/Report_English-2.pdf.
[b] Bank for International Settlements (BIS). 2020. Annual Report Economic Report 2020. https://www.bis.org/publ/arpdf/ar2020e1.pdf.
[c] ADB. 2021. COVID-19 and the Finance Sector in Asia and the Pacific. https://www.adb.org/sites/default/files/institutional-document/761946/covid-19-finance-sectorasia-pacific-guidance-note.pdf.
[d] The Geneva Association. 2021. Public-Private Solutions to Pandemic Risk: Opportunities, Challenges and Trade-Offs. https://www.genevaassociation.org/sites/default/files/research-topics-document-type/pdf_public/pandemic_solutions-report_final.pdf.

3.   **The different nature of the financial impact of disasters triggered by natural hazards and long-lasting epidemics and pandemics requires differing financial instruments and enabling measures.** Figure 1 illustrates the different timeline and impacted areas by disasters and pandemics and epidemics.

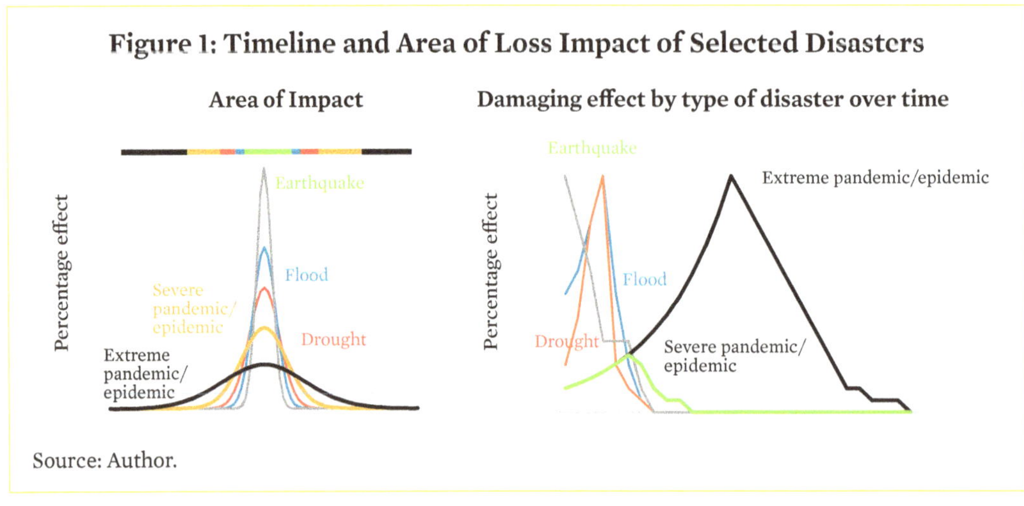

Figure 1: Timeline and Area of Loss Impact of Selected Disasters

Source: Author.

4.   **Enhanced financial preparedness for disasters is an Asian Development Bank (ADB) priority.** The ADB technical assistance (TA) project, *Strengthening the Enabling Environment for Disaster Risk Financing (Phase 2)* under which this document is prepared, is consistent with ADB's 2021 Disaster and Emergency Assistance Policy, which explicitly supports enhanced financing arrangements for disasters, epidemics, and pandemics (ADB 2020). It is also consistent with the Financial Sector Directional Guide under development by ADB, which calls for building capabilities in emerging and innovative finance areas such as DRF.

5.   **ADB's holistic approach to DRF is reflected in this TA.** ADB strongly advocates an integrated approach to disaster risk management, seeking to strengthen disaster resilience both through disaster risk reduction and the enhanced management of residual risk. ADB is seeking to enhance financial preparedness for disasters as part of broader efforts to strengthen disaster resilience. It is doing so in close coordination with governments, global and regional DRF initiatives,[1] standard-setting bodies (International Association of Insurance Supervisors), International Organization of Securities Commissions, the Basel Committee on Banking Supervision, the Islamic Financial Services Board, the Financial Stability Institute), and the insurance industry. Disaster risk reduction efforts should be the first consideration in addressing disaster risk, tackling the root causes of the issue. DRF solutions should also conform to international financial standards and be designed around the context of broader disaster resilience, financial stability, and financial inclusion, incorporating incentives for disaster risk reduction. This approach should lead to the development and implementation of financially sustainable, scalable DRF strategies, and solutions. ADB applies a risk layered approach to support the appropriate selection of disaster risk management options, including DRF instruments (section 1.2).

6.   **This country diagnostics assessment identifies areas that can be improved to enhance the enabling environment for DRF in the Kyrgyz Republic.** Notwithstanding the importance of having and using DRF instruments, these instruments can only be fully effective under certain conditions that are often neglected. Assessing and identifying barriers to be removed to create an enabling environment for increased uptake of these instruments is critical. This country diagnostics is intended to facilitate the development and implementation of appropriate instruments for different layers of risk. It identifies areas of improvement to enhance the enabling environment for public sector DRF solutions as well as insurance, reinsurance, and capital market (IRCM) solutions.

7.   **Recommendations based on the assessment are comprehensively presented in the corresponding sections.** The recommended activities and measures to enhance the enabling environment for key public sector DRF instruments, as well as IRCM solutions, are presented at the end of the corresponding section. The main recommendations are also summarized in the executive summary.

---

[1] The Vulnerable Twenty Group; the Disaster Risk Financing and Insurance Program of the World Bank, Market Global Practice and Global Facility for Disaster Reduction and Recovery; and the Pacific Disaster Risk Financing and Insurance Program; and the Asia-Pacific Economic Cooperation and the Organisation for Economic Co-operation and Development promoting the G20/OECD Methodological Framework for Disaster Risk Assessment and Risk Financing.

1.2   Risk Layering Approach

8.   **Resilience begins with risk reduction, that is, acting to reduce levels of loss in the event of natural hazards, epidemics, and pandemics.** However, risk cannot be eliminated, so investments in financial preparedness need to be enhanced to ensure sufficient financing to support timely relief, early recovery, and reconstruction efforts.

9.   **Governments can draw on an array of instruments to enhance financial preparedness.** These instruments are ideally applied using a risk layering approach, breaking risk down according to the frequency of occurrence of different types of hazard events, epidemics, and pandemics of varying severity and associated levels of loss and designing bundles of instruments targeting differentiated layers of risk (ADB 2013). Governments should select the most appropriate instruments for each layer of risk based on a range of factors, including scale of funding needed, speed of disbursement required, and relative cost-effectiveness of alternative instruments for specific layers of risk. Due to the unexpected severity of COVID-19 pandemic, most financing instruments used were ex post; and to support the financial sector, regulatory forbearance was necessary (Box 2).

**Box 2: Policy Measures Taken for the Financial Sector
to Combat COVID-19 Pandemic**

In response to the coronavirus disease (COVID-19) pandemic, the National Bank of the Kyrgyz Republic postponed the enactment of several financial regulations until further notice (March 2023). It also (i) lowered the liquidity ratio (ratio between liquid assets and liabilities) to a minimum of 30% (from the current 45%); (ii) removed liquidity ratio requirements (7-day and overnight/instant); (iii) reduced the minimum threshold for mandatory reserve requirements from 80% to 70%; (iv) reduced risk weights of foreign exchange for corporate and retail loans from 150% to 100%; (v) called for banks and nonbank financial institutions to create a loan–loss reserve equal to 100% for the amount of overdue accrued interest payments on loans given the status of non-accrual of interest income when overdue arrears are 270 days or more (from 90 days); and (vi) stated that , in the event of arrears arising from the COVID-19 pandemic, banks or nonbank financial institutions have the right to not downgrade the classification category due to financial condition of the borrower. Commercial banks can delay or restructure payments of the principal of loans extended to business and people for 6 months, if desired by borrowers.

Source: International Monetary Fund. 2021. *Policy Reponses to COVID-19.* https://www.imf.org/en/Topics/imf-and-covid19/Policy-Responses-to-COVID-19.

10.   **DRF instruments for residual risk begin with risk retention instruments for more frequent, less damaging events (Figure 2).** These include annual contingency budget allocations, reserves, and contingent grant and credit arrangements, all of which are put in place before an event strikes. After an event, governments can also reallocate budgets, increase borrowing, and raise taxes to provide additional resources.

11.   **Market-based risk transfer solutions provide more cost-efficient financing for medium-level risks, generating higher levels of loss but less frequently.** These include insurance and insurance-linked securities, such as catastrophe bonds, and are taken out in anticipation of potential disasters, epidemics, or pandemics. Following major events, governments also appeal to the international community for assistance.

12.   **DRF is not only a government responsibility; the private sector and individuals should be encouraged and enabled to share in this.** A similar risk layering approach is applicable. Decisions on risk reduction, retention, and transfer should be made within the structure of this broader framework, selecting appropriate instruments for each layer of risk. The insurance sector is called to play an important role in this by developing tailor-made products suitable to the Kyrgyz Republic.

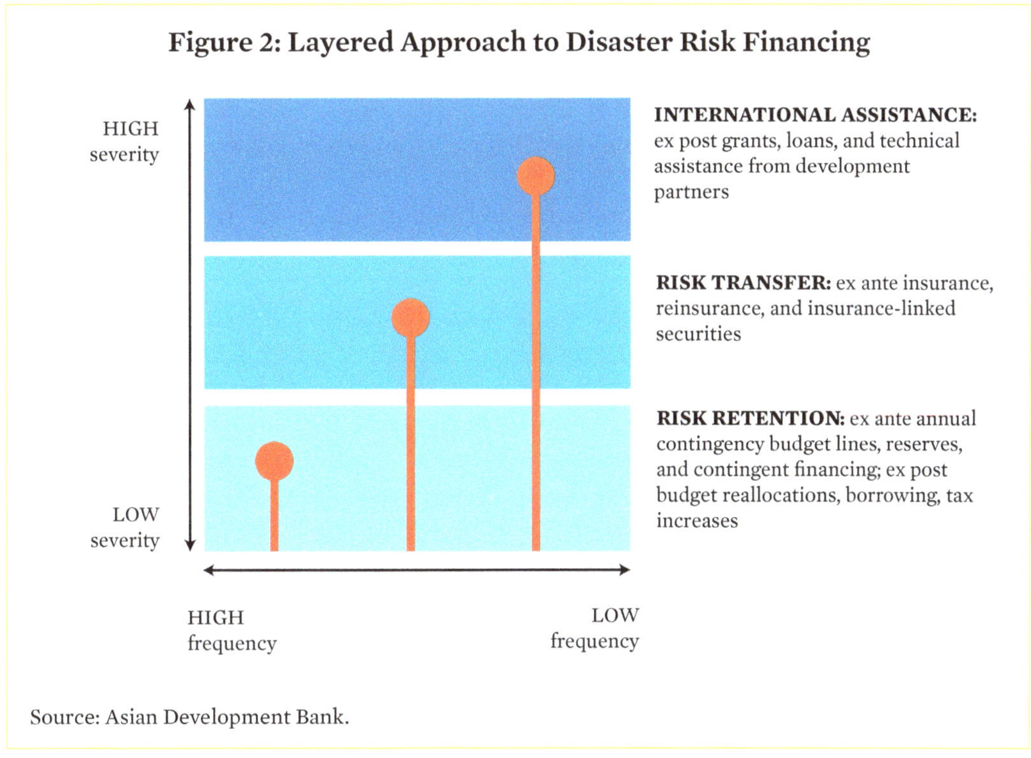

Source: Asian Development Bank.

13.   **The availability and assortment of instruments selected for a DRF strategy depend on a range of factors.** The most appropriate bundle of instruments depends on the scale of resources required at each layer of loss relative to the scale of resources each instrument can facilitate access to; the speed with which funds are required relative to the disbursement speed of each instrument; the marginal cost of each instrument; individual country circumstances, including prevailing macroeconomic circumstances; the scale of potential events relative to gross domestic product (GDP); government economic, fiscal, and monetary goals and objectives; access to international finance markets; and the market-based cost of borrowing (ADB 2013). For example, if probable maximum losses from extreme events are low relative to GDP, then a country is better able to retain risk. A country with low indebtedness can rely more on post-event borrowing than one with a higher level. The effectiveness of risk transfer instruments also depends crucially on the availability of well-developed and sound domestic insurance and capital market sectors. Among other issues, the cultural and religious dimensions are important, and notably, government policy could potentially crowd out the private insurance sector.

1.3 Diagnostics Methodology

1.3.1 Diagnostics Tool

14.   **The country diagnostics have been undertaken applying a diagnostics tool developed and used for the assessment of four other countries under phase 1 of this TA.** However, the tool has been enhanced to cover the assessment of the enabling environment for pandemic and epidemic risk financing instruments.

15.   **The diagnostics tool covers sovereign and nonsovereign risk financing instruments.** Governments apply risk financing instruments to protect their budgets. Governments can also provide an adequate enabling environment to encourage the supply and uptake of nonsovereign insurance, such as homeowner and commercial property insurance, business interruption cover, health insurance, and crop insurance. In the process, they can reduce the contingent liability falling on government.

16.   **The diagnostics tool generates an overview of current policies and mechanisms for DRF.** It identifies enabling conditions for the effective use of well-established DRF instruments, the introduction of new instruments and related barriers and gaps; sets policy priorities for implementing reforms and introducing new DRF instruments; and provides the basis for new or deeper engagement on DRF by governments, regulators, and development partners as part of broader disaster, epidemic and pandemic risk management and public financial management dialogue. The findings of the diagnostics can feed directly into the development of strategies to enhance the financial risk management of disasters, pandemics, and epidemics.

17.   **The tool includes two structured questionnaires.** The first questionnaire helps assess the framework used by the government to finance disasters, epidemics, and pandemics within its budget, i.e., when disaster risk is retained. The second questionnaire provides insights on risk transfer instruments. The two questionnaires are critical for evaluating the existing enabling environment for both risk retention and risk transfer instruments.

18.   **The assessment of the enabling environment for the effective use of risk retention instruments is based on a joint ADB and World Bank (2017) questionnaire.** The questionnaire has been enhanced to include epidemic and pandemic risk financing (Box 3).

19.   **The assessment of the enabling environment for the effective use of disaster risk transfer instruments is based on a modified version of the "W&W Development Framework."**[2] This framework was refined to provide a methodology for assessing the DRF landscape and its enabling environment. It focuses on six areas of relevance for the development of disaster, epidemic, and pandemic IRCM solutions as follows:

- **Economic conditions and other support functions,** such as the disposable budget for insurance, the level of indebtedness. It also includes data availability, financial sector specialized courts and health facilities, doctors, vaccines and epidemic and pandemic research institutes, risk managers, insurance, and other relevant professionals (e.g., actuaries, adjustors, accountants) for the well-functioning of IRCM providers.

---

[2] The W&W Framework has been used on several occasions by Rodolfo Wehrhahn, one of the assessors, to determine barriers to an enabling environment in work done for ADB, the International Monetary Fund, and the World Bank. The relevant areas for an enabling environment as determined in this framework follow from Wehrhahn (2010).

Box 3: Examining the Full Sovereign Disaster Risk Finance Landscape

The Asian Development Bank–World Bank disaster risk financing diagnostic assesses sovereign financial protection against disasters. It has been extended in this report to include questions for ministries of health and of finance. It includes questions pertaining to risk transfer sovereign arrangements but has a strong focus on risk retention mechanisms. The questions cover the following issues:

The assessment of fiscal shocks associated with disasters, epidemics and pandemics impacting the:

i.   contingent liability of the government
ii.   fiscal risk assessment of disaster, epidemic, and pandemic shocks; and
iii.   public disclosure of fiscal exposure to disasters, epidemics, and pandemics.

Ex ante risk financing instruments

i.   annual contingency budget
ii.   dedicated budget lines for risk reduction
iii.   dedicated reserve funds
iv.   line agency funding
v.   contingent credit and grant arrangements
vi.   insurance of public assets
vii.   other forms of sovereign insurance
viii.   risk transfer arrangements through capital markets

Ex post risk financing instruments

i.   Post-event budget reallocations
ii.   External assistance
iii.   Tax increments
iv.   Government borrowing

Source: Adapted from ADB and the World Bank. 2017. Assessing Financial Protection against Disasters: A Guidance Note on Conducting a Disaster Risk Finance Diagnostic.

- **Government policy on the development of risk transfer instruments.** This includes the introduction of mandatory insurance protection, risk-pooling structures, and insurance-linked securities,[3] pertinent regulations, and a level playing field for IRCM activities.
- **Credibility of the private sector offering risk transfer solutions.** This covers issues such as the regulatory environment, the solvency of risk carriers, the reputation of insurance and capital markets. It also covers the professionalism of distribution channels, loss adjusters, brokers, and the availability of infrastructure (e.g., stock exchanges, payment systems, etc.).

---

[3] Insurance-linked securities bonds, including catastrophe bonds and other risk-linked securitization, represent assets whose value is largely driven by the occurrence of events not correlated to the financial markets, allowing for a high degree of diversification. With an insurance-linked securities bond, the investor is exposed to a well-defined catastrophic or insurable event in addition to the credit risk of the issuer. For this additional exposure, investors are compensated with higher coupons, but if no covered event occurs during the risk period the bonds are redeemed at 100% of face value. When a covered event meets the thresholds in the risk transfer contract, investors stand to lose coupon payments and/or a percentage of the principal. The redemption price of the bonds is reduced accordingly. For more details, see ADB (forthcoming).

- **Disaster and epidemic and pandemic risk product availability and affordability.** This includes products for governments, corporates, small and medium-sized enterprises, farmers, individual households, and low-income population.
- **Social protection policy.** Low-income populations should enjoy social protection and at least basic health protection or support in obtaining insurance coverage, while insurance solutions for people that can afford the premiums should not be crowded out. This should also explore the degree to which social protection complements or might be crowding out market-based solutions.
- **Unlicensed competition.** The resilience of insurance providers depends on adequate oversight. Unlicensed entities or those poorly supervised by agencies with insufficient insurance supervision and risk management expertise can destroy the image of insurance and leave consumers without protection should a disaster cause their insolvency.

20.   **The Toolkit for Insurance, Reinsurance and Capital Market Solutions for Disaster Risk Financing, revised version (ADB, forthcoming), presents a fuller description of the tool, including the two questionnaires.** The document presents a generic tool kit for disaster, epidemic and pandemic, and IRCM solutions and focuses on actions to strengthen the enabling environment to support DRF instruments, including a glossary of technical terms.

1.3.2 Application of the Diagnostics Tool

21.   **The diagnostics tool is used to determine and confirm DRF practices and gain insight into existing or perceived barriers hindering the development of DRF instruments.** The tool is applied through a combination of desk-based work, stakeholder questionnaires, interviews, and group discussions. This wide-ranging approach is taken to accommodate international good practice of countries with successful results and draw in expert judgment on actions needed to better enable effective DRF mechanisms.

22.   **The basic steps are as follows:**

- As a starting point, background information on the DRF strategy of the focus country is gathered. The information is drawn from extensive publications, government documents and websites, insurance and reinsurance industry documents, and capital market analyses.
- The background information is then complemented with extensive questionnaires with open questions on areas relevant to the DRF approach and instruments used in the country. These questionnaires, integral to the diagnostics tool, are sent to relevant stakeholders for their inputs. The insights gained are critical for a robust assessment, and questions to the stakeholders are explained carefully, stressing the importance of providing comprehensive and open answers.
- On-site interviews take place with selected stakeholders from both the public sector and IRCM stakeholders, including actuaries, rating agencies, brokers, and auditing firms. These interviews enhance and complete the information gathered through the desk analysis and the questionnaire responses.
- The comprehensive information is then analyzed and gaps between international good practice and current practices are identified.

- The recommended actions are discussed with the stakeholders and the feasibility and relevance confirmed before the country diagnostic is finalized.
- Implementation of the recommendations should follow.

23.   **Stakeholders are not necessarily expected to respond to all questions.** Experience shows that the questionnaire will provide wide-ranging responses, including contradictory statements, and leave some questions unanswered. The assessors review and filter the information to draw preliminary conclusions. These conclusions are then verified with stakeholders repeatedly before finalizing the findings and recommendations.

1.3.3 Presentation of the Diagnostic Results

24.   **The country diagnostic reports begin by presenting the findings to the broad public sector DRF landscape, including related recommendations.** The results of the diagnostic analysis are then presented and finally summarized in a spider diagram depicting country scoring for each of the six areas of relevance for the development of a strong enabling environment for disaster and epidemic and pandemic IRCM solutions (Figure 3). For each area, an ideal, a realistic, and the current state of the environment are depicted.

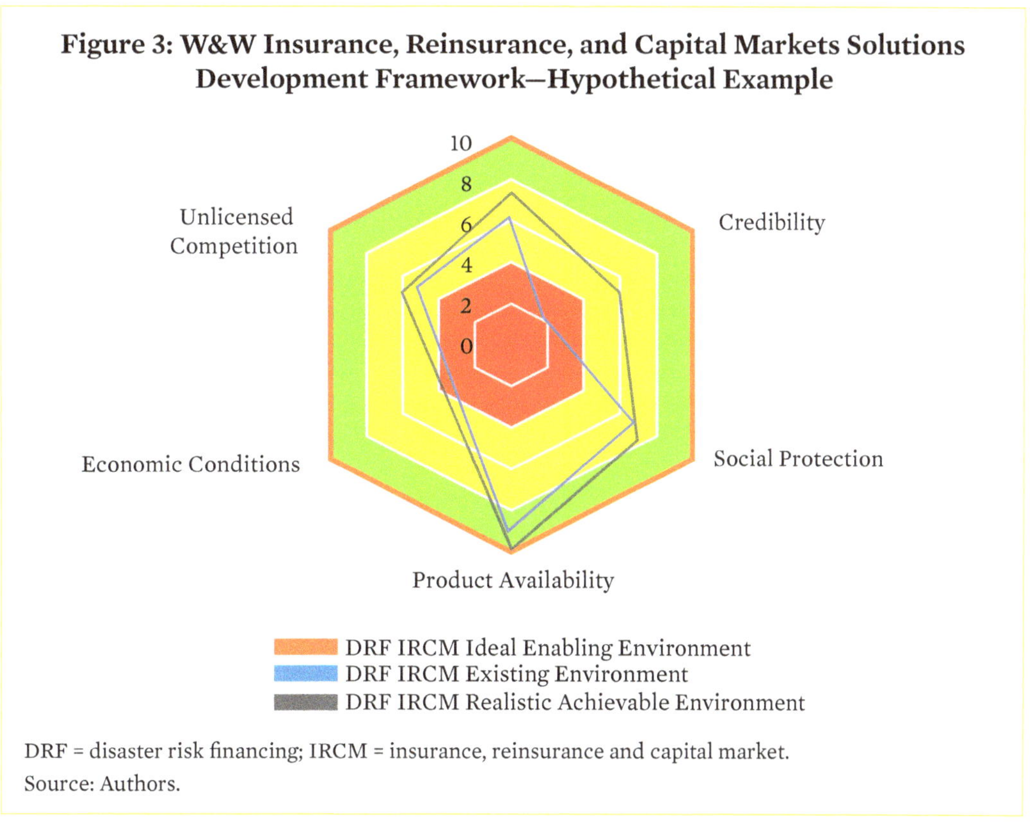

Figure 3: W&W Insurance, Reinsurance, and Capital Markets Solutions Development Framework—Hypothetical Example

DRF = disaster risk financing; IRCM = insurance, reinsurance and capital market.
Source: Authors.

25.   **The ideal enabling conditions for the development of IRCM solutions for each of the six areas are defined.** The assessors define this environment based on international good practice and expert judgment. This step considers the political, cultural, and religious contexts of the marketplace as well as international best practice.

26.   **A reality check defines the next best IRCM solutions enabling environment that can be achieved.** The ideal enabling environment may be very difficult to achieve in practice and, as such, a realistic enabling environment for each of the six areas is determined on a country-by-country basis. This is the best achievable enabling environment and is developed drawing on local expertise gained through extensive stakeholder consultation and analysis of the questionnaires to identify likely impediments to this achievement. The ideal and realistic enabling environments will not necessarily differ significantly and, thus, may overlap.

27.   **The current environment is then populated.** Using local expertise and comments from relevant national stakeholders, including government authorities, private sector providers, and professional bodies, the current environment for each of the axes is determined.

28.   **The methodology used, thus, depicts the gaps between the current enabling environment for disaster IRCM solutions and the ideal and realistic alternatives.** The comparison enables ready identification of areas for action, leading to the development of a strategy and road map for the removal of the gaps. The prioritization of actions to address the gaps should be based on the scale of the gap and reflect reasonable time frames for completion. Urgent actions are recommended to strengthen the enabling environment in relevant areas achieving scores of four or below (color red), medium-term actions are recommended for scores between four and six (yellow), and no immediate actions are required for higher scores (green). Where the realistic enabling environment differs from the ideal scenario, that difference between the existing and the realistic scenario rather than between the existing and the ideal scenario is considered when determining the urgency of the needed actions. The absolute scores have no further meaning and should not be used for cross-country comparisons.

Public Sector Disaster Risk Financing Landscape

2.1 Background

29.   **The Kyrgyz Republic is located in a seismically active and mountainous region and exposed to a wide range of natural hazards.** According to the Ministry of Emergency Situations, the country faces around 20 types of hazards. The most frequent and damaging are earthquakes, floods, landslides, mudslides, avalanches, snowstorms, mountain lake spills, droughts, and epidemics. The country is located between the Tian Shan and the Pamir mountains, with 40% of it above 3,000 meters, over 80% within the Tian Shan mountain range, and 4% permanently covered in ice and snow (World Bank and ADB 2021). The majority of the population (7 million)[4] live in the foothills of the two mountain ranges. As such, earthquakes, floods, and landslides along mountain rivers, triggered by heavy rainfall and rapid snowmelt, affect a significant proportion of the population and cause considerable economic damage (CAREC Program 2022a). In particular, earthquakes have caused loss of life, destroyed homes, and ruined livelihoods. On 5 October 2008, for instance, an earthquake measuring 8 points on Richter scale destroyed most houses and killed 74 in Nura village in Osh region. Box 4 details those and other damages from major disasters. While earthquakes caused more economic damage than any other disaster during the 1991–2021 period, floods and landslides have been the most frequent disaster events.

30.   **Table 1 shows key disaster-related statistics for the Kyrgyz Republic.** Disasters affected 2,275,962 people and caused over $404 million in reported damage during the period. Earthquakes impacted 176,063 people and caused a reported damage of over $328 million. Floods and landslides affected 89,839 people and caused total reported damage of over $67 million. A major drought in 2009 affected 2 million people.

31.   **While low-intensity disasters are common in the Kyrgyz Republic, Box 4 details the human and economic losses of major earthquakes, landslides, and floods.**

32.   **Since economic loss data is not available for all reported disasters—recorded in EM-DAT during 1991–2020—which result in actual losses were likely significantly higher.** According to the Central Asia Regional Economic Cooperation (CAREC) Program, for instance, the average annual modeled loss from floods in the Kyrgyz Republic is estimated to be over $73 million and that from earthquakes at around $72 million, which results in a combined annual average loss of more than $145 million (CAREC Program 2022b). CAREC estimates show the average number of people severely affected by floods every year is 4,400 and earthquakes at 5,570. Figure 4 depicts exceedance probability curves for flood and earthquake risk in the Kyrgyz Republic. According to World Bank estimates, average annual losses from disasters amount to nearly $270 million ($200 million in damages

---

[4]   National Statistical Committee of the Kyrgyz Republic.

Table 1: Key Natural Disaster Statistics (1991–2021)

Year	No. of People Affected by Each Disaster Category[a]						Total Deaths	Total Damage ($ '000)
	Earthquake	Landslide	Epidemic	Flood	Drought	Storm		
1992	86,806						54	251,047
1992	50,000						4	59,856
1994		58,500					111	65,811
1994							51	
1997	1,230							3,376
1997			336				22	
1998				7,728			1	3,990
1998			458					
2002		1,002						2,260
2003		211					38	
2004		309					49	
2005				2,050			3	3,691
2006						9,075	4	
2006		12,050						
2007				845				261
2008	4,197						74	
2009					2,000,000			
2010			8,350					
2010	141							
2012				11,000				
2015	16,780							13,719
2017	5,000							
2017		55					24	
2021		15						
Total	164,154	72,142	9,144	21,623	2,000,000	9,075	435	404,011
Percentage	7%	3%	0.40%	1%	88%	0.4%		

[a] Damage and loss data for some disaster events are not reported in the EM-DAT database, and this table does not include data on COVID-19 pandemic.

Source: EM-DAT, the International Disaster Database. https://www.emdat.be (accessed 13 March 2022).

from earthquakes, $60 million from floods, and $2.6 million from landslides) (World Bank 2018a), or over 3.5% of GDP.[5] It estimates disasters affect around 280,000 people annually (Burunciuc 2020).

33.   **The COVID-19 pandemic took a severe toll on people and the economy.** The World Health Organization (WHO) says there were 206,399 confirmed COVID-19 cases and 2,991 deaths in the country.[6] From 2019 to 2020, the percentage of people living in poverty increased from 20.1% to 25.3%.[7] About 60% of the population lived on less than $5.5/day prior to the

---

[5]   This calculation includes the average of GDP for five pre-pandemic years during 2015–2019.

[6]   Taken from the WHO COVID-19 Dashboard, Kyrgyzstan COVID-19 Situation. https://covid19.who.int/region/euro/country/kg.

[7]   National Statistical Committee of the Kyrgyz Republic. http://www.stat.kg/en/opendata/category/120/ (accessed 8 December 2022).

Box 4: Major Disaster Events

On 5 October 2008, an earthquake measuring 8.0 in magnitude on Richter scale, destroyed most houses in the village of Nura, in the Alay district of Osh region. It caused 74 deaths, including 32 preschool and 12 older children, in a settlement of just 900 people.[a]

In 1998, severe floods on Kurgart River led to a river dam breach, which destroyed 1,199 houses and caused an estimated $134 million in direct damages.[b]

In April 1994, massive landslides and debris flows caused by torrential rains affected over 58,000 people, led to 111 deaths, destroyed 520 houses, and made 13,200 people homeless.[c]

On 19 August 1992, a strong earthquake of magnitude 7.5 on the Richter scale occurred in the Toluk region, near the country's border with the People's Republic of China. It affected an estimated 146,900 people, caused 75 deaths, and incurred damage of $237 million (in 2019 prices).[d][e]

Sources:

[a] Reliefweb. 2008. Kyrgyz Quake Raises Questions over Shoddy Buildings. 17 October. https://reliefweb. int/report/kyrgyzstan/kyrgyz-quake-raises-questions-over-shoddy-buildings.

[b] CAREC. Country Risk Profile, Kyrgyz Republic. https://www.carecprogram.org/uploads/CAREC-Risk-Profiles_Kyrgyz-Republic.pdf.

[c] Asian Disaster Reduction Center (ADRC). Kyrgyz Republic. https://www.adrc.asia/nationinformation. php?NationCode=417&Lang=en&NationNum=28.

[d] WFP. Logistics Capacity Assessment. Kyrgyz Humanitarian Background. https://dlca.logcluster.org/ display/public/DLCA/1.1+Kyrgyzstan+Humanitarian+Background.

[e] Central Asia Regional Economic Cooperation (CAREC). Country Risk Profile, Kyrgyz Republic. https://www.carecprogram.org/uploads/CAREC-Risk-Profiles_Kyrgyz-Republic.pdf.

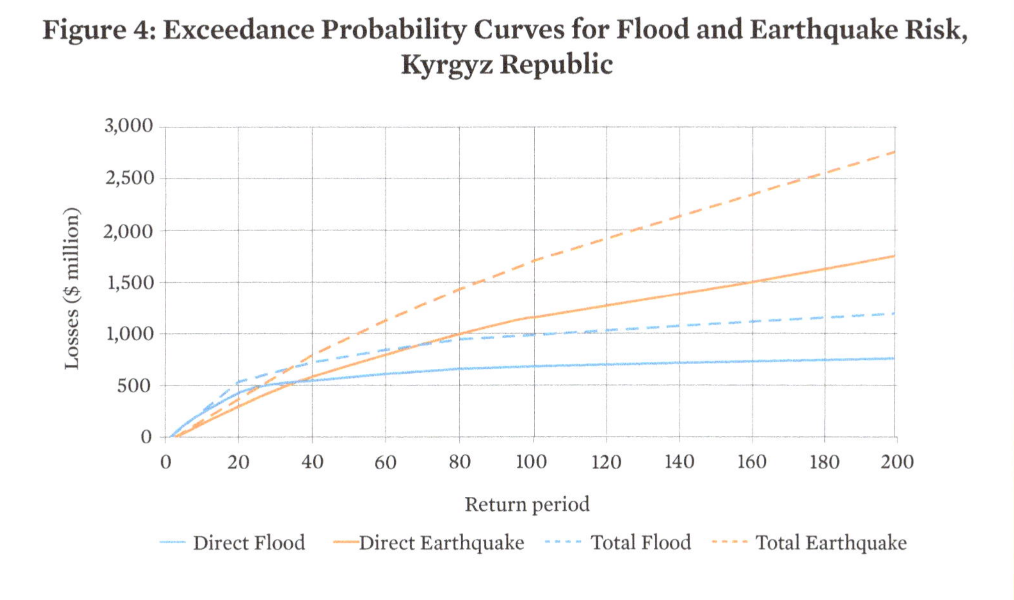

Figure 4: Exceedance Probability Curves for Flood and Earthquake Risk, Kyrgyz Republic

Source: Central Asia Regional Economic Cooperation (CAREC) Program. 2022a. *Country Risk Profile, Kyrgyz Republic, CAREC Secretariat.*

pandemic (IMF 2021a). Unemployment increased from 6.9% in 2019 to 9.1% in 2021.[8] World Bank estimates suggest that poverty level may have increased to 38% in 2022 (World Bank 2022). GDP contracted 8.4% in 2020, after expanding by 4.6% in 2019—a steep 13 percentage point decline.[9] In 2020 alone, the country spent over $560 million in its response—reaching 7.2% of GDP in 2020 and leading to an increase in public debt by 16.5% of GDP (IMF 2021b). The government has not indicated how much it received in total assistance from development partners. However, public data indicate over $800 million was approved in grants and loans (Table 3).

34.   **Disaster loss models project devastating human and economic losses from infrequent but severe disaster events.** Disaster loss models by CAREC show that less frequent but more severe earthquake and flood events could cause high economic losses. For instance, losses from a 1-in-100-year combined earthquake and flood event could be over $1.8 billion. That is, an earthquake event alone could cause $1.16 billion in economic loss, or 18.6% of the country's GDP; while a flooding event could lead to $680 million in losses, or about 8% of GDP (CAREC Program 2022a). Earthquake event loss scenarios project even more devastating casualties and damage to private and public infrastructure assets in the Kyrgyz Republic (Free, Coates, and Fourniadis 2018). Based on their model, expected (mean) earthquakes with magnitude of 7.5 (moment magnitude scale) in the Ferghana Valley (return period of 475 years)—predominantly affecting the region near the cities of Jalal-Abad and Osh—could cause fatalities "over 5,500 in residential buildings, over 7,500 in school buildings as well as over 150 direct casualties in hospital and fire station buildings." The associated monetary losses are expected to be (i) over $6 billion to residential buildings; (ii) around $300 million to transport infrastructure (roads and bridges); and (iii) hundreds of millions of dollars to schools, hospitals, and other buildings. The authors also project that an earthquake of similar magnitude on the Issyk-Ata geological fault occurring near Bishkek is likely to result in similar fatalities and economic losses. The World Bank in 2017, using a probabilistic and scenario-based seismic hazard and risk assessment,[10] put estimated economic losses to residential buildings "when subjected to scenario earthquake shaking results" as high as $16 billion, with fatalities as high as 19,000 people (World Bank 2017). These models do not include projection of human and economic impact of pandemics. The COVID-19 virus outbreak reminded the world that infectious diseases can spread fast and easily across countries and cause severe human and economic impact. It is therefore essential that country-specific pandemic impact models, once developed, are considered to assess overall pandemic impact.

35.   **The country's financing needs to build climate resistance infrastructure—including replacing existing dated infrastructure—remain among the highest in the region.** A significant share of infrastructure is left over from the Soviet Union era and is thus vulnerable to natural hazards. To address infrastructure challenges and build climate-resilient infrastructure, the country increased public investment in infrastructure from 4.8% of GDP in 2011 to 7.6% in 2015 (OECD 2019). According to the United Nations Economic and Social Commission for Asia and the Pacific (UNESCAP), infrastructure investments amounted to about $14 billion during 2000–2018, where more than 50% of investments were directed to energy projects and

---

close to 40% to transport (UNESCAP 2021). However, UNESCAP estimates a financing gap in transport, energy, and information and communication technology for 2018–2030 at about 19% of the country's GDP (UNESCAP 2021). The transport sector, where road transport accounts for 95% of all traffic in the country, is in dire need of financing. According to the Organisation for Economic Co-operation and Development (OECD), existing road capacity (rehabilitation of existing and construction of new roads) would need to increase by 251% by 2030 and by an overwhelming 985% by 2050 to meet the country's upcoming needs and reduce the very high transport costs. Further, "[a]bout 45 percent of the capital assets used for power generation are beyond their useful life, and in the distribution system, electricity towers and underground cables are in urgent need of replacement" (World Bank 2020).

36.   **Infrastructure maintenance is weak and enforcement of building regulations, primarily from a seismic safety perspective, is limited.** Due to shortages in road maintenance funds, for instance, one-third of the country's 35,000 kilometer road network is in poor condition (Holzhacker and Skakova 2019). According to the World Bank, since the 1990s, substantial reduction in investment and operation and maintenance budgets for irrigation systems has led to the deterioration of the country's irrigation infrastructure. Also the country's aging energy infrastructure system's wear and tear is assessed at over 50%, also due to inadequate investment (IEA 2020). In addition, over 80% of public school buildings and structures are highly vulnerable to natural hazards, according to UNICEF, as they do not meet safety requirements and are in dire need of retrofitting, repair, and reconstruction. Moreover, poorly constructed private houses, particularly in the remote areas, are highly vulnerable to earthquakes—mainly from a seismic safety perspective (Box 4). In addition, "larger settlements and even recently-built housing estates in urban areas are just as likely to collapse in the event of a big quake" (Reliefweb 2008).

37.   **Climate change stresses such as increases in temperature, greater frequency and intensity of extreme weather events, and glacial melt may amplify disaster-induced risks in the Kyrgyz Republic.** The country was ranked 75th out of 181 countries in the 2020 ND-GAIN Index. The ND-GAIN Country Index summarizes a country's vulnerability to climate change and other global challenges in combination with its readiness to improve resilience (University of Notre Dame 2020). The Kyrgyz Republic considers its water, energy, agriculture, and infrastructure sectors as the most vulnerable to climate change. These climate change priorities are identified in the country's strategic documents, such as the National Development Strategy of the Kyrgyz Republic for 2018–2040, and the Climate Investment Program of the Kyrgyz Republic and Program for the Development of a Green Economy in the Kyrgyz Republic for 2019–2023. Average annual temperature in the Kyrgyz Republic reaches around 2°C, with high elevation areas experiencing temperature below –20°C. While temperatures in the summer occur in the high tens to low twenties, they regularly exceed 30°C from June to August in the lowland regions (World Bank and ADB 2021). Climate change scenario analyses show temperature in the Kyrgyz Republic may rise significantly above the global average, "warming over the 1986–2005 baseline period could reach 5.3°C by the 2090s, under the highest emissions pathway" (World Bank and ADB 2021). Modelling projects a 4°C rise in temperature in the country is likely to cause the GDP to contract by 1.5% (Kompas, Pham, and Che 2018). In addition, average annual precipitation in the country is 389 millimeters (mm), ranging from 300 mm in the eastern parts of the country to 600 mm in the southern.[11] Climate change projections suggest precipitation in the north-east of Osh region is likely to increase to double that of the mean annual, while southern regions could receive up to 20% more (CAREC Program 2022a). According to CAREC, "Osh and the capital

---

[11] United States Agency for International Development (USAID). Climate Change Analysis for the USAID/Kyrgyz Republic, 2020–2024 CDCS. https://www.climatelinks.org/sites/default/files/asset/document/2021-07/2021_USAID_CDCS-Annex-Kyrgyz-Republic.pdf.

city Bishkek are projected to have significant intensification, with what used to be the 1 in 100-year events becoming the 1 in 50-year events by the 2050s" (CAREC Program 2022a). Climate change models suggest higher temperatures are likely to accelerate the country's glacier melt. Glaciers in the Northern Tian Shan decreased an average of 25%–30% between 1955 and 1999.[12] Acceleration in glacier melt is likely to (i) intensify river runoff and increase risks of severe flood and landslide events, amplifying their already high human and economic impact; (ii) lead to decline in water availability in the long run; and (ii) heavily impact the country's agriculture sector and hydroelectric generation on which it is highly dependent. Agriculture, for instance, employs 31.7% of the country's workforce and depends on water from seasonal glacier runoffs, and the hydroelectric power plants supply 87% of the Kyrgyz Republic's electricity (OECD 2019). Furthermore, as part of the Central Asia–South Asia power project (CASA-1000), the Kyrgyz Republic and Tajikistan are to supply electricity to Afghanistan and Pakistan—completion expected in 2023. The 1,400-kilometer project—dependent on water from seasonal glacier runoff—is considered a significant new source of revenue for the two countries, and is expected to transmit 4.6 billion-kilowatt hours/year.[13]

38.   **The country, with support from development partners and global research institutions, has improved its weather forecasting and seismic earthquake early warning services.** The National Meteorological and Hydrological Service (KyrgyzHydromet), as well as the Ministry of Emergency Situations, under which it operates, "follows a value chain approach, where local monitoring is combined with satellite data and global forecasts to inform national models" (Kull, Jukusheva, and Naqvi 2022). The government utilizes this mechanism to forecast weather at regional and local levels and inform local authorities of possible disaster events in advance, such as storms and floods. In 2014, the first real-time digital strong-motion network in Central Asia was installed in the country—for earthquake early warning and rapid response (Parolai et al. 2017). With support from development partners and global research institutions, the country has improved its early warning capabilities. Teaming up with the GFZ German Research Centre for Geosciences Kyrgyz, in 2020, the country developed a real-time dam monitoring system that senses "vibrations, ground movements and long-term structural deformations of the structures" (GFZ Helmholtz Centre Potsdam 2020). The system provides early warnings from earthquakes and is even able to provide damage forecasts.

39.   **While the Kyrgyz Republic has improved its weather forecasting and seismic earthquake monitoring capability to identify areas prone to natural hazards—fiscal risk analyses are lacking.** In October 2020, the full registration of the government's nonfinancial assets was completed, except for subsoil assets. According to the country's 2021 Public Expenditure and Financial Accountability (PEFA) performance assessment, a detailed presentation of the government's fiscal risks is included in the Explanatory Notes of the Republic Budget, primarily in terms of "adverse external economic developments reducing revenue and adding to the burden of external debt" (PEFA 2021). As well, the annual Republic Budget includes provision for dealing with emergencies arising from floods and landslides (PEFA 2021). However, the explanatory notes do not seem to include details on exposure of public assets to disasters and, most importantly, quantification of the government's fiscal risks arising from disasters.

---

[12] USAID. Climate Change Analysis for the USAID/Kyrgyz Republic, 2020–2024 CDCS.
[13] CASA-1000. *CASA-1000: Increasing Clean Energy Availability and Access in Central and South Asia.* https://www.casa-1000.org/#:~:text=The%20%241.2%20billion%20CASA%2D1000,kilowatt%20hours%20 (kWh)%2Fyear.

2.2 Institutional Disaster Risk Management Arrangements

40.   **The overall disaster risk management system in the Kyrgyz Republic includes a range of regulations, a national strategy, and institutional arrangements, encompassing disaster response at the national, regional, local, and object levels—including epidemics and pandemics.** In January 2020, in response to the COVID-19 pandemic the government established a special coordination center under the Office of the Prime Minister. Key regulations guiding the overall management of disasters include the following:

- The Decree of the Kyrgyz Republic "On protection of population and territory from natural and man-made emergency," approved in 2000.
- Decree No. 746 "On the Unified State Emergency Preparedness and Response System," endorsed on 23 October 2006.
- Decree No. 175 "On the Ministry of Emergency Situations of the Kyrgyz Republic," endorsed on 16 May 2007.
- Law on International Disaster Relief, adopted in June 2017, governing international humanitarian assistance during large-scale disaster emergencies.
- Law No. 45 on Civil Protection, adopted on 24 May 2018, which "regulates legal relations arising in the field of civil protection of the population and the territory of the Kyrgyz Republic in emergency situations in peace and wartime."[14]
- Concept of comprehensive protection of the population and territory of the Kyrgyz Republic from emergencies for 2018–2030 was approved by the Decree of the Government of the Kyrgyz Republic dated January 29, 2018 No. 58. Action plan to implement the concept of comprehensive protection of the population and territory of the Kyrgyz Republic from emergency situations for 2018–2030 (stage 2, 2023–2026) has been developed and yet to be approved (UNDP 2022).

41.   **The National System of Civil Protection is responsible for protecting the people of the Kyrgyz Republic as well as its territories during emergencies.** The system manages and resources a wide range of local and state agencies, local branches of national emergency institutions, nongovernment organizations, and other voluntary organizations.[15] The government provides civil protection services to the affected population during disasters through relevant regional and city branches of central institutions. Under the leadership of the Prime Minister, the Inter-Ministerial Commission of Civil Protection coordinates the National System of Civil Protection at the national level.[16] Its members include Inter-Agency Commission members, cabinet ministers, heads of government agencies, and heads of regional administrations and cities.

---

[14] FAOLEX Database. https://www.fao.org/faolex/results/details/en/c/LEX-FAOC196590/ (accessed December 2022).

[15] WFP. Kyrgyzstan Humanitarian Background. https://lca.logcluster.org/11-kyrgyzstan-humanitarian-background.

[16] Anticipation Hub. *Kyrgyzstan. Key Facts.* https://www.anticipation-hub.org/experience/anticipatory-action-in-the-world/kyrgyzstan#:~:text=The%20Ministry%20of%20Emergency%20Situations,their%20aftermath%20in%20the%20country.

42.   **The Ministry of Emergency Situations serves as the operational branch of the government and the primary working body of the National System of Civil Protection.** The Minister of that ministry serves as the first deputy of Inter-Ministerial Commission of Civil Protection. The ministry also serves as the overall operational body for the special coordination center established under the Office of the Prime Minister in response to COVID-19. The ministry provides organizational and technical support to the Inter-Ministerial Commission of Civil Protection and serves as the Secretariat to the Inter-Ministerial Commission for Elimination of Natural Disasters, a high-level body consisting of various government institutions. As the overall national disaster risk management coordinating body, the ministry coordinates activities—disaster risk reduction, emergencies, and early and post recovery—with other central agencies, territorial governments, local authorities, donor partners, as well as local and international nongovernment organizations. Its main objectives include

- forecasting of natural and man-made hazards and planning civil protection measures;
- warning and implementing preventive measures against peace and war time emergencies; and
- search, rescue, early recovery, and other urgent operations, elimination of emergency consequences, and impact assessment.[17] Post-disaster reconstruction activities are carried out by relevant central agencies, and state and local governments.

43.   **During disasters, the Ministry of Emergency Situations works with civil defense, other central agencies, territorial governments, and local authorities to assess damage and subsequently mobilize resources.** As an independent budgetary unit, the ministry receives annual budget allocation for its operations ($5.0 million–$5.6 million annually). The ministry also has access to disaster contingency funds, discussed in the following section. Figure 5 depicts the ministry organization structure.

44.   **The ministry cochairs the seven sector groups under the Disaster Response Coordination Unit.** The unit is a consultative coordinating body consisting of development partners (donor community, nongovernment organizations, the Red Crescent, and the UN agencies). The aim of the unit is to enhance coordination between the government and its development partners in disaster response.

---

[17] WFP. Kyrgyzstan Humanitarian Background. Logistics Capacity Assessments. DLCA-1.1KyrgyzstanHumanitarian Background-090522–0321–3452.pdf.

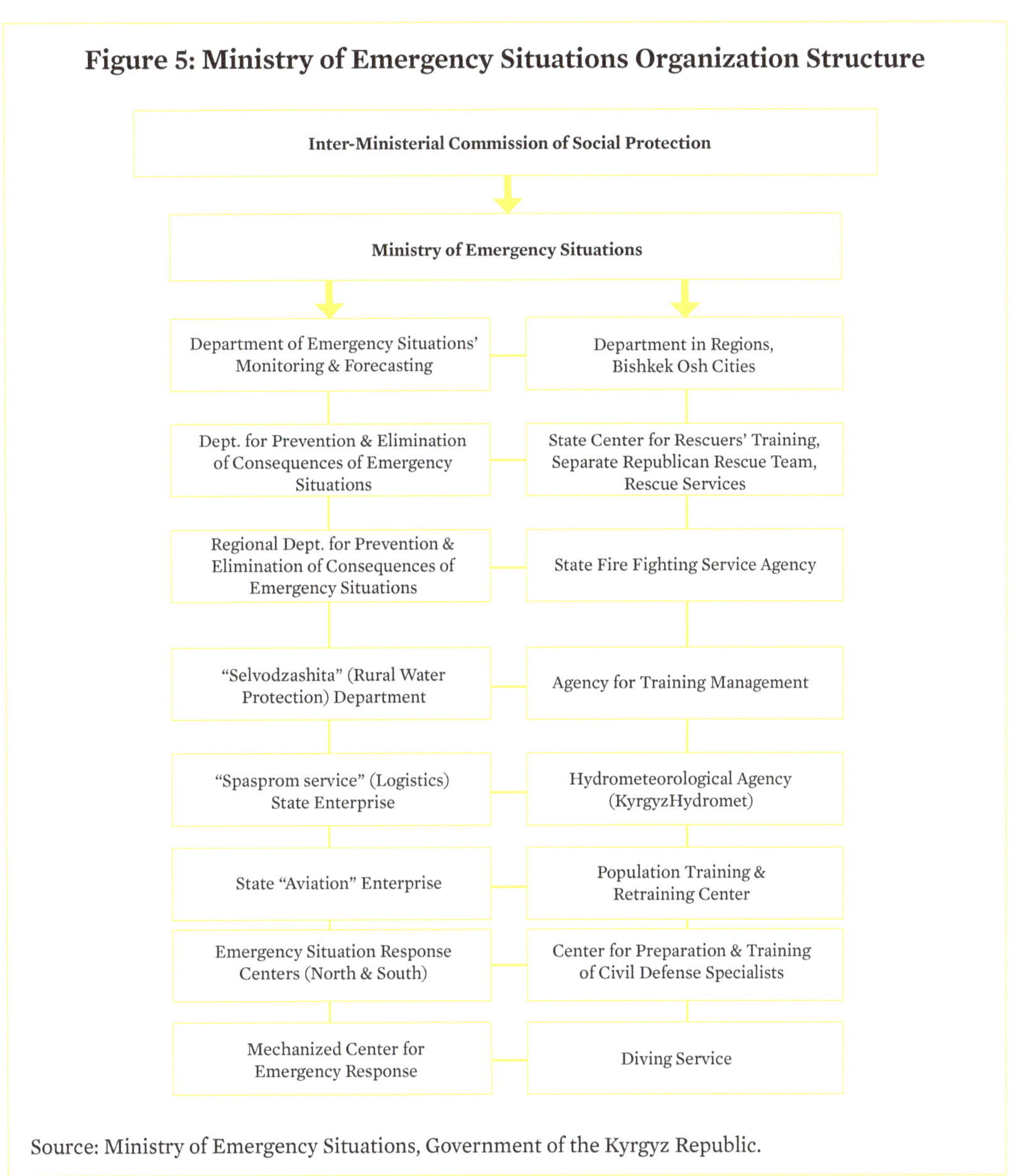

Source: Ministry of Emergency Situations, Government of the Kyrgyz Republic.

2.3 Disaster Risk Financing Mechanisms and Instruments

45. **Post-disaster-related expenses in the Kyrgyz Republic are funded mostly through the sovereign DRF instruments outlined in the sections below.** Except for mandatory disaster home insurance,[18] most such expenses are funded through the Republic Budget.

---

[18] More information on disaster home insurance is provided under the Social Protection section.

2.3.1 Ex Ante Disaster Risk Financing Mechanisms

46.   **Disaster emergencies in the Kyrgyz Republic are first funded through the Ministry of Emergency Situations budget.** As Table 2 shows, approved Republic Budget, including special funds of the ministry, amounted to Som3 billion ($37.7 million) in 2022. The ministry's expenditures during fiscal year (FY) 2021 were Som2.722 billion ($34.24 million), and Som1.9 billion ($23.93 million) in FY 2020. According to the ministry, about Som400 million–Som450 million ($5.00 million to $5.67 million) of its approved annual budget is allocated to the ministry's operating expenditure. The remainder is set aside for disaster response and, subsequently, distributed across local governments and line ministries at the beginning of the fiscal year based on the government's risk assessment—using a weather monitoring approach in coordination with relevant government agencies to identify regions at potential risk. Municipalities also allocate small funds (between Som100,000 and Som1 million) for disaster emergencies from their own resources based voluntarily. Additionally, according to the Ministry of Finance, the Ministry of Emergency Situations in 2022 has access to Som7 billion ($88 million) emergency reserve fund that it can use to respond to disaster emergencies, early recovery, and rehabilitation. Furthermore, if required, state reserve funds (reserve and other funds of territories)—amounting to Som2.9 billion in 2022 approved budget, or $36.5 million—can also be accessed to fund disaster response. Therefore, when the ministry spends its approved budget, it can request more funds through the Ministry of Finance from the mentioned funds. Available funds for disasters in 2022—Ministry of Emergency Situations approved budget, emergency and reserve funds—accounted for around 4% of the total approved 2022 national budget. Allocation of the emergency and state reserve funds to state and local agencies, coordinated by the Ministry of Finance, requires the approval of the Cabinet of Ministers and a budget committee of Parliament. According to the 2020 Public Expenditure and Financial Accountability (PEFA) assessment, however, the government makes minimal use of its contingency reserves. "Emergency funds made up less than 0.15% of total budgeted expenditure in 2017–2019" (PEFA 2021). The low utilization of emergency funds in recent pre-pandemic years seem to be due to low damage caused by disasters. Furthermore, according to the Ministry of Finance, following the pandemic, the government has created a $250 million Stabilization Fund to respond adequately to emergencies. However, it is unclear how the fund is resourced and how much of the resources can be used for disaster emergencies, rehabilitation, and reconstruction.

Table 2: Ministry of Emergency Situations Republic Budget

Currency	2020 Total Expenditures (million)	2021 Total Expenditures (million)	2022 Total Approved (million)
Kyrgyz Republic som	1,902	2,722	3,010
United States dollar	23.93	34.24	37.86

Source: Ministry of Finance, Kyrgyz Republic.

47.   **Disaster recovery and reconstruction activities are first funded through the annual Ministry of Emergency Situations budget.** Subsequently, line ministries, agencies, and local governments are encouraged to use their allocated budgets to fund the mentioned activities. When they exhaust their allocated budgets, line ministries, agencies and local

governments can request more funds through the Ministry of Finance—which, in turn, submits these requests to the Cabinet of Ministers and a budget committee of Parliament for approval. According to the line ministries, however, most of their disaster-related funding needs in recent years have been met through the Ministry of Emergency Situations budget.

2.3.2　Ex Post Disaster Risk Financing Mechanisms

Budget Reallocation

48.　**Line ministries, agencies, and local governments utilize their allocated budgets to respond to disaster recovery and reconstruction only when the approved Ministry of Emergency Situations budget is exhausted.** Therefore, in recent years, these institutions rarely needed to reallocate significant portions of their allocated funds to respond to disaster recovery and reconstruction. According to line ministries, when they need to reallocate their budgets to respond to disasters, their requests to the Ministry of Finance are normally approved in full and within a short time, while requests for additional resources are assessed and approved based on availability of resources at the national level.

2.3.3　External Assistance and Financing

49.　**The Kyrgyz Republic relies on official development assistance (ODA) to fund its development priorities.** During 2015–2020, according to the OECD Creditor Reporting System database, disbursed ODA to the country amounted to $5.3 billion, or about $528 million per year on average.[19] Grants during this period accounted for 79% of total disbursed ODA, and loans for the remaining 21%. ODA during this period amounted to nearly 8% of the GDP. The government has access to lending instruments (loans and grants) to fund disaster-related expenses—donor support during the COVID-19 pandemic is a recent example. The government has not provided a figure for the total support it received from development partners related to the COVID-19 pandemic. However, as noted, publicly available data compiled for this report show development partners approved over $800 million in external assistance to the country in response to COVID-19 (grants and loans) (Table 3).[20]

50.　**Development partners provide humanitarian assistance in response to disasters.** While the Government of the Kyrgyz Republic does not keep records of humanitarian assistance, as this is delivered directly to beneficiaries, humanitarian assistance plays a pivotal role in the country's overall disaster risk management. As indicated under section 2.3, while disaster risk management funding in recent years in response to minor events came mostly from the government's budget, donor partners also provide humanitarian support during disasters. According to the OECD Creditor Reporting System database, the country received about $30 million in humanitarian aid and $5 million in emergency response during 2012–2020. Of this amount, the country received over $19 million in 2019 and 2020, likely in response to COVID-19 pandemic. International aid is expected remain available, and the country is familiar with the administration of those funds, and as such, no recommendation on those instruments is necessary.

---

[19] OECD. Creditor Reporting System. https://stats.oecd.org/Index.aspx?DataSetCode=crs1 (accessed December 2022).

[20] Actual assistance may be higher as these figures may not include assistance from all development partners, the total figure includes both disbursed and committed assistance.

Table 3: External COVID-19 Support, Commitments, and Disbursements

Donor	Amount ($ million)
International Monetary Fund	242.00
Asian Development Bank	228.43
World Bank & Asian Infrastructure Investment Bank	150.00
World Bank	88.00
European Union	42.00
German Development Bank KfW	30.00
Islamic Development Bank	15.00
United States Agency for International Development	10.00
Total	805.40

COVID-19 = coronavirus disease.

Source: Donors' websites.

2.3.4 Diagnostic and Recommended Actions

51.   **Existing budget allocations are sufficient to enable the government to retain fiscal shocks arising from annual disaster events.** With the exception during the COVID-19 pandemic, when the government tapped into its emergency and reserve funds, disaster-related expenses in recent years have been funded mostly through the Ministry of Emergency Situations budget—about $32 million (net of operating expenses) on average during 2019–2022. According to CAREC, average annual "modelled loss" from floods and earthquakes in the Kyrgyz Republic amounted to about $146 million (CAREC Program 2022a). Therefore, total available government resources of $160 million (Ministry of Emergency Situations as well as contingency and reserves) seem sufficient to finance average annual losses from disasters (under normal circumstances).

> *Explore options for securing a contingent disaster financing facility. As indicated above, existing public resources are limited—close to 9% of projected loss from infrequent but severe disaster events. Therefore, following the risk layered approach, the government may seek to establish contingent disaster facilities with support from development partners. Such a funding mechanism will enable quick access to budget support that the country could draw on following qualifying disaster events. This would help enable the government to manage fiscal shocks arising from disasters without stretching existing limited sovereign resources or potentially delaying maintenance of infrastructure and implementation of ongoing and planned public investment projects and social programs.*

52.   **The financing of infrequent but severe disaster events needs attention.** For instance, the CAREC disaster risk model predicts losses from a 1-in-100-year combined earthquake and flood event that could be over $1.8 billion. In contrast, based on existing budgetary allocations, the government has access to about $160 million to respond to disasters, close to 9% of the projected losses from infrequent but severe disaster events. Based on figures given earlier, this includes the Ministry of Emergency Situations annual budget and special

accounts ($37.7 million in 2022), primary funds used to respond to disasters; state emergency funds not earmarked for disasters ($88 million); and reserve funds also not earmarked for disasters ($36.5 million). These projections do not include the economic impact of pandemics. It is, thus, essential to consider country-specific pandemic impact models, once developed, to assess overall impact of disasters.

> ***Acquire risk transfer solutions for the disaster events of medium severity and frequency.*** *Following the risk layer approach, these type of events are better financed with a combination of sovereign insurance, reinsurance, and capital market solutions.*

53.   **However, there is limited information on the exposure of public assets to disasters and, more importantly, the quantification of the government's fiscal risks resulting from such events.**

> ***Enhance the collection of information and related analysis regarding fiscal risks arising from disasters.*** *Government incorporates various fiscal risk scenario analyses in its annual budget planning. These analyses should be based on past disaster events (including the COVID-19 pandemic) and future ones to assess related contingency liability. Resulting lessons should be used to enhance fiscal management of disaster risk.*

Diagnostic on the Current Availability and Utilization of Insurance, Reinsurance, and Capital Markets for Disaster Risk Financing

3.1 Economic Conditions and Other Support Functions

3.1.1 Economic Landscape

54. **Following a significant COVID-19 pandemic-induced contraction, the Kyrgyz Republic's economy has begun a gradual rebound, as noted in para 33.** The government, with support from development partners, responded swiftly to mitigate the pandemic's impact on public health and the economy. According to the International Monetary Fund (IMF), these measures included emergency health spending, a food security program, temporary tax deferrals and subsidized loans to small and medium-sized enterprises, liquidity support to banks, deferrals of loan payments, and temporary relaxation of capital and loan provisioning norms. These amounted to 7.2% of gross domestic product (GDP) ($560 million) in 2020 and led to an increase in public debt from 16.5% of GDP to 68% (IMF 2021).

55. **Remittance inflows, accounting for 31.3% of GDP, fell significantly in US dollar terms due to the COVID-19 pandemic and international sanctions on the Russian Federation following its invasion of Ukraine, resulting in a steep decline in the ruble against the US dollar.** The Kyrgyz Republic's economy is highly sensitive to external shocks, due to its heavy dependence on remittances, export of goods and services (35.23% of GDP), and import of goods and services (64.14% of GDP).[21] Over a million Kyrgyz nationals live and work in the Russian Federation, the country's main trading partner. Remittance inflows accounted for 31.3% of Kyrgyz Republic GDP,[22] while remittances from the Russian Federation ($2.7 billion) accounted for nearly 80% in 2021 (Lillis 2022). Due to rising food prices, and a temporary decline in remittance inflow in the initial stage of the Russian invasion of Ukraine, people living under the poverty line increased to 38.0% in 2022, from 21.1% in 2020 (World Bank 2022).

56. **Economic growth was projected to slow down to 3.8% in 2023 from 6.3% in 2022, and recover slightly to 4% in 2024 if external events were not prolonged (Figure 6).** Inflation remained high at 15% in 2022 and 12% in 2023, mainly from a more than 20% surge in fuel and gas prices that may push up prices of food and other items. Inflation is projected to decline to 8.6% in 2024.

---

[21] World Bank. World Integrated Trade Solutions. https://wits.worldbank.org/CountryProfile/en/KGZ#:~:text=Kyrgyz%20Republic%20exports%20of%20goods,percentage%20of%20GDP%20is%2064.14%25.

[22] World Bank. Data. https://data.worldbank.org/indicator/BX.TRF.PWKR.DT.GD.ZS?locations=KG.

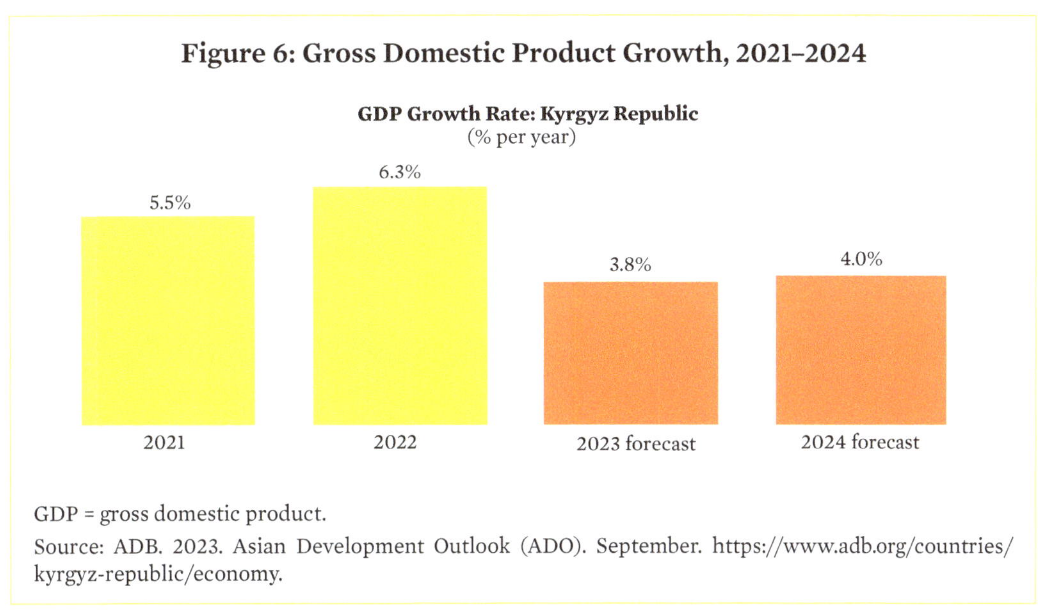

GDP = gross domestic product.
Source: ADB. 2023. Asian Development Outlook (ADO). September. https://www.adb.org/countries/kyrgyz-republic/economy.

57.   **The government recognizes both short- and long-term socioeconomic implications of external events and disasters, including pandemics.** The government created a \$250 million Stabilization Fund to respond adequately to emergencies, says the Ministry of Finance. However, it is unclear how the fund would be financed and whether the resources can be used for non-pandemic disaster emergencies, rehabilitation, and reconstruction. The Ministry of Finance also indicated that the government is looking forward to the recommendations of this report in terms of securing resources from development partners to respond adequately to natural hazards.

3.1.2   Insurance Support Functions

58.   **The country lacks insurance professionals to support the 17 active insurers.** Only companies with foreign capital have access to actuaries and underwriters, limiting the ability to provide proper pricing, reserving and development of insurance products. The insurance regulator does not have an actuary in its staff and thus its capacity to assess the technical soundness of the insurance sector is restricted.

3.1.3   Pandemics and/or Epidemics Support Functions

59.   **The health system suffers from human resource shortages (Figures 7, 8, and 9).** As of 2019, the Kyrgyz Republic had 219 physicians and 397 nurses per 100,000 population, both below the average for Central Asia. The health workforce is very unevenly distributed between urban (Bishkek and Osh) and rural areas. Some rural areas have only 70 physicians per 100,000 population (1 physician per 1,249 people). In contrast, hospital beds stand at 407 per 100,000 population, having decreased from more than 700 in 2000 (even higher than the European Union average), but still considered at overcapacity inherited from the Soviet Union era.[23]

---

[23] Hydrometeorological Service, Ministry of Emergency Situations of the Kyrgyz Republic. http://meteo.kg/

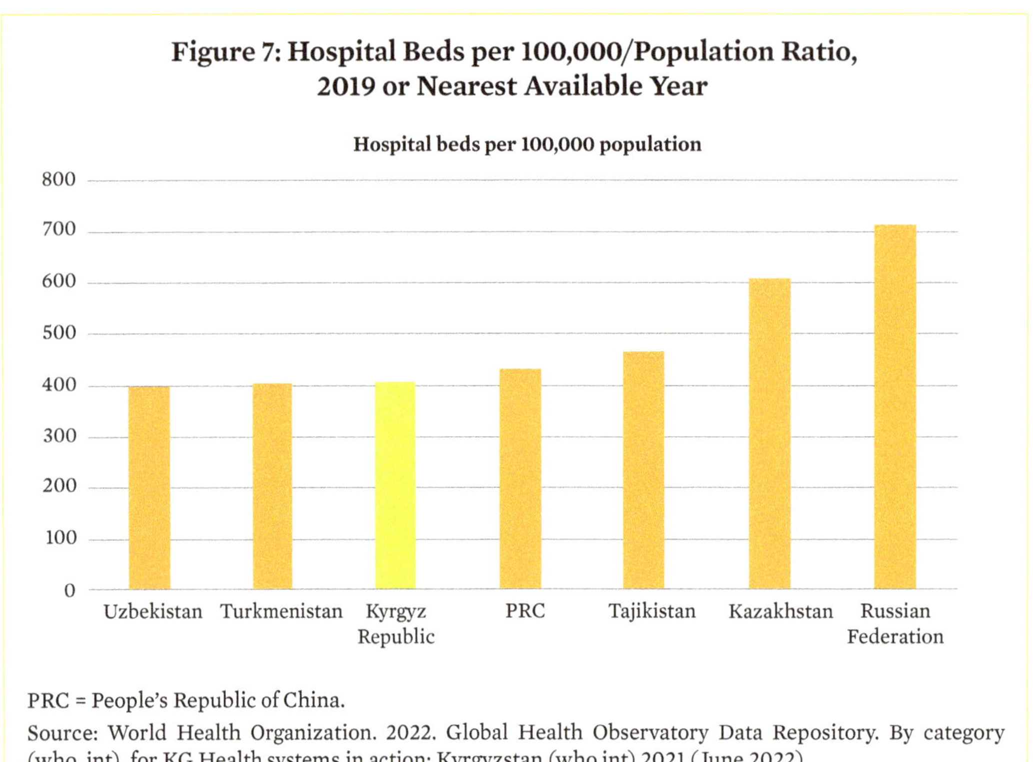

Figure 7: Hospital Beds per 100,000/Population Ratio, 2019 or Nearest Available Year

PRC = People's Republic of China.

Source: World Health Organization. 2022. Global Health Observatory Data Repository. By category (who. int), for KG Health systems in action: Kyrgyzstan (who.int) 2021 (June 2022).

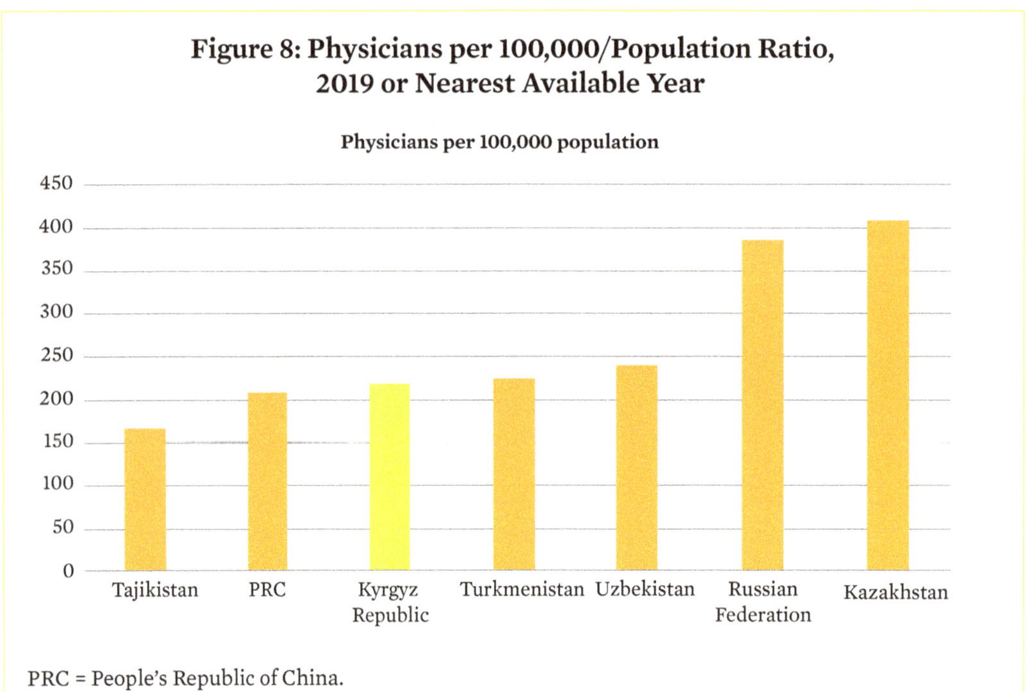

Figure 8: Physicians per 100,000/Population Ratio, 2019 or Nearest Available Year

PRC = People's Republic of China.

Sources: World Health Organization. Global Health Observatory data repository. GHO | By category (who.int) (accessed June 2022); for Kyrgyz Republic, European Observatory on Health Systems and Policies. Health Systems in Action: Kyrgyzstan (who.int) 2021 (accessed June 2022).

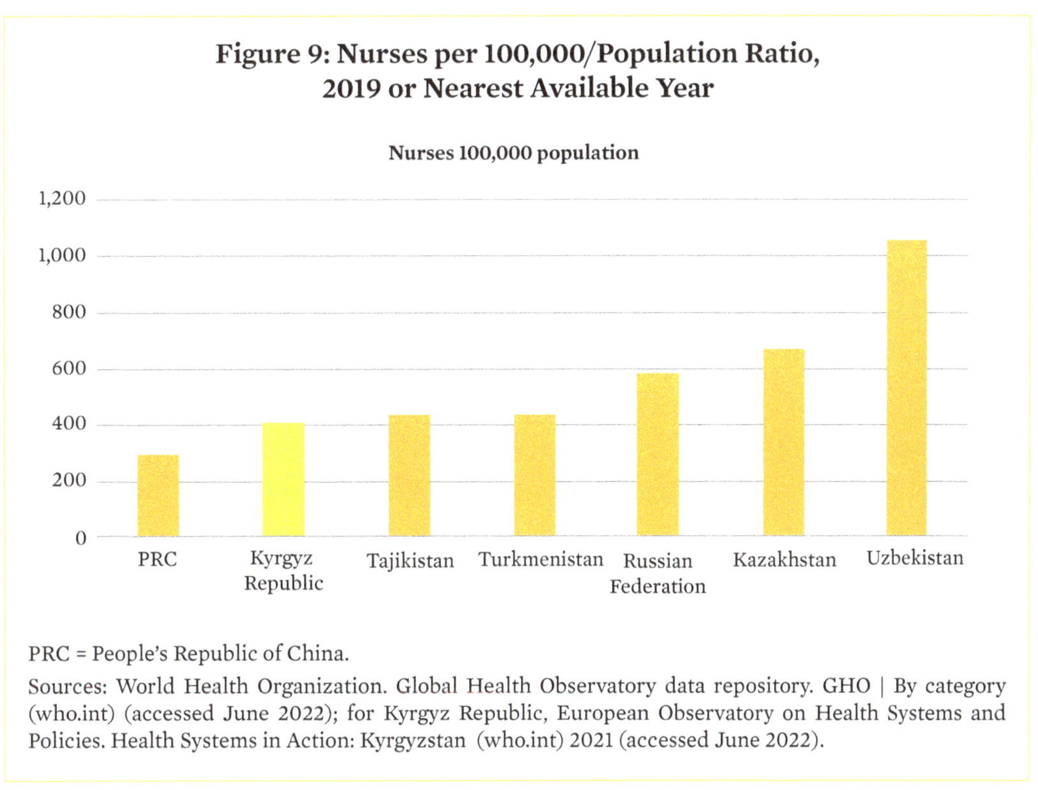

PRC = People's Republic of China.

Sources: World Health Organization. Global Health Observatory data repository. GHO | By category (who.int) (accessed June 2022); for Kyrgyz Republic, European Observatory on Health Systems and Policies. Health Systems in Action: Kyrgyzstan (who.int) 2021 (accessed June 2022).

3.1.4 Agriculture Insurance Supporting Meteorological Infrastructure

60. **The Hydrometeorological Service of Kyrgyz Republic was established in 1926.** The main tasks include systemic observation of meteorological, hydrological, agrometeorological, and other conditions. The service collects and analyzes data and produces weather forecasts and various analytical reports. It is guided by the framework of the Word Meteorological Organization to the United Nations and the Interstate Council for Hydrometeorology of The Commonwealth of Independent States (CIS).[24]

61. **The service operates different types of observation locations and equipment located throughout the country.** These include traditional ground-based manual weather stations; automated weather stations; automatic sensors; hydrological and agrometeorological posts; snow, air, and water quality observation posts; etc. It planned to deploy an additional 24 automatic weather stations in 2022 in cooperation with the World Bank.[25]

62. **The Hydrometeorological Service offers a variety of forecast and analytical reports, including 10 days and monthly agrometeorological reports and phenological data for farmers.** Most historical weather data are in hard copy. Weather data in e-format is available starting in 2015.[26] The service can provide historical weather data on demand to any customer but it is a paid service, with the Ministry of Agriculture as the main customer.

---

[24] Hydrometeorological Service. http://meteo.kg/.

[25] Based on notes from the meeting with the Hydrometeorological Service management during a virtual mission in May 2022.

[26] This information was provided by the Hydrometeorological Service during the virtual meeting in May 2022.

3.1.5 Data Availability

63.   **Historic data is not readily available, both at the aggregated and granular levels which are necessary to develop and design suitable DRF instruments.** While a number of probabilistic disaster risk models have been constructed with the support of development partners and research institutions[27] in recent years, there has been "an almost complete lack of official data from the relevant authorities (e.g., roads from the Ministry of Transport, school buildings from the Ministry of Education, etc." (World Bank 2017).

64.   **Various health information systems in place are currently not integrated.** Data from primary health care are collected through the national electronic database for such care administered by the Ministry of Health's eHealth Center. Secondary and tertiary level data are reported to the Mandatory Health Insurance Fund under the ministry. In parallel, other data bases and reporting systems exist (e.g., for vaccination), which are not integrated. The Ministry of Health coordinates data reporting. As these databases do not use a unique identifier for patients and are technically not compatible, further consolidation of the data is hampered. Data entry at primary health care is entered monthly into the system, often manually, which makes the data more error-prone and creates a systematic delay in data availability. No dedicated disease outbreak warning system is in place (Laatikainen et al. 2022; WHO 2018a, 2020). According to the National Development Plan, 2022–2026, the government plans to digitalize the COVID-19 surveillance system.

65.   **The Kyrgyz Republic has the basic data needed for agriculture insurance, but scope exists for improvement.** This includes the following weather and agriculture production data:

- *Weather data.* Historical weather data is available from the Hydrometeorological Service, but much work is needed to become effective for assessing agriculture risk. This government agency accumulates data including meteorological, hydrological, agrometeorological, environmental, and others.
- Since 2010, the Hydrometeorological Service has deployed 57 automatic weather stations within the framework of various projects (e.g., World Bank), which were acquired through a different tendering process. As a result, the network is not homogeneous, but sensor types seem to be comparable. Data quality management for automatic weather stations seems to be limited to factory standards, presumably gross error checks. No additional downstream quality control procedures are applied either to check the validity of the data or to detect technical problems with the individual stations. For traditional manual stations, observers do manual quality control and consistency checks at a purely IT level are done automatically (Alliance for Hydromet Development and World Bank 2021).
- The Hydrometeorological Service provides raw data (and forecasts, warnings, crop yields, and phenological forecasts) to sectoral users including the Ministry of Agriculture. No open government data policies are in place. National legislation requires the service to charge a fee for the provision of weather and other data.
- *Production data.* Agriculture production data is available at the National Statistical Committee of the Kyrgyz Republic.[28] Such data that are open to the public includes

---

[27] The ADB/CAREC model was developed by Willis Towers Watson.
[28] National Statistical Committee of the Kyrgyz Republic. Agriculture. http://www.stat.kg/en/statistics/selskoe-hozyajstvo/ (accessed 15 August 2022).

area planted, harvested, crop yields, volume of production, livestock, etc., which is the basic data required for agriculture insurance. Publications and spreadsheets at the National Statistical Committee website confirm that data is available at the *raion* (district) administrative level, which could be used for initial rate setting, underwriting, and product development.

- *Insurance data.* Such data, including loss ratios and premium charged, is not available at the insurance regulator. This is because agriculture insurance is not recognized as a separate insurance class or sub-class and insurance companies are not required to provide data for this type of insurance (see paras. 125–126 on agriculture insurance). Currently, agriculture insurance data (premium, number of policies, number of claims, and claims sums) are reported under the fire risk class and these do not provide reliable data to analyze the status of agriculture insurance in the country.

3.1.6   Diagnostic and Recommended Actions

66.   **The lack of insurance professionals limits the ability of insurers to develop disaster risk insurance products.** The shortage needs to be addressed.

> ***Establish a strategy to develop insurance professionals.*** *Working together with the regulator, the industry should develop a medium-term strategy to develop key professionals to support the development of the insurance sector. Studying the insurance professionals development strategy in place in Kazakhstan could be useful in this context.*

67.   **Investments in weather monitoring infrastructure are insufficient.** Disaster risk management in agriculture requires huge weather infrastructure, such as automatic weather stations, hydrometeorological stations, doppler radars, moisture sensors, satellite imagery, drones, and mobile applications. The data and insights generated through this infrastructure is critical for disaster risk reduction and DRF.

> ***Increase investment in weather infrastructure to support disaster risk financing mechanisms.*** *While the market for such data remains limited, the government will have to lead investment in weather infrastructure. However, as the utility of accurate weather data coupled with analytics through artificial intelligence and machine learning expands to a variety of players such as banks, insurance/reinsurance companies, agriculture research institutions, exporters, importers, etc., the investment program in weather infrastructure can be transformed into a public–private partnership initiative.*

68.   **Substantial agritech progress in other countries has led to smarter insurance products to protect the livelihoods and incomes of farmers.** Essentially, agritech solutions can enhance farm-level risk management, risk reduction, risk monitoring, yield estimation, and loss assessment. Not just insurers, but also farmers, lending institutions, agri-input providers, traders, economists, climate scientists, policymakers, and agriculture researchers can benefit significantly from agritech. Globally, many technological interventions for agriculture are being designed and implemented. These include:

- *Robots and smart appliances.* Companies are developing and programming autonomous robots to handle essential agriculture tasks such as sowing seeds and harvesting crops at a higher volume and faster pace than human laborers. This is addressing the problem of availability, productivity, and high cost associated with agriculture labor.

- *Crop and soil monitoring.* Companies are leveraging computer vision and deep-learning algorithms to process data captured by drones and/or software-based technology to monitor crop and soil health. The outputs include advisories on optimal use of soil nutrients, fertilizers, and pesticides. These applications enable farmers to improve productivity.
- *Predictive analytics.* Machine learning models are being developed to track and predict environmental impacts on crop yield, such as weather changes. These analytics are used to alert farmers of adverse weather conditions well in advance, optimal sowing and harvesting periods, possible pest attacks, etc.
- *Specialized farming chatbots such as Alexa are being developed to assist farmers in their day-to-day issues.* Farmers can get customized advice from remotely located experts by sharing ground-level information through photographs on a range of issues.
- *Crop loss assessments through satellite imagery, drones, and ground-level data retrieved from mobile applications.* These can enable lending institutions and insurance companies to assess losses accurately and quickly, for timely payment of claims.
- *Market information and access through mobile applications.* These enable farmers to assess future commodity prices and adjust their crop selection. Applications also link farmers to agriculture markets and potential buyers, enabling them to get the best price for their produce without having to deal with intermediaries

Develop agritech to reduce risk to a level where insurance becomes sustainable and affordable.

69.   **The availability and access to disaster risk models provides the basis for a robust DRF strategy and the pricing of insurance premiums.** Notwithstanding that the country is highly exposed to major disasters, availability of risk data, hazard models, and historical losses and damage records does not exist at a sufficiently granular level.

Collect necessary data from the relevant government ministries on disaster events affecting the country

Develop an open source disaster risk model covering all major hazards, including pandemics/epidemics faced by the country.

70.   **The existing health information landscape and pandemic surveillance data systems are still fragmented and partly manually operated.** During the COVID-19 pandemic, the country set up an on-time reporting system for case reporting and hospitalization; however, these were temporary and would have to be reactivated in a new pandemic. This leads to lack of availability of on-time information.

Develop and implement a health information systems integration strategy. This will increase the robustness of pandemics/epidemics-related data availability throughout the health system, including permanent systems for on-time pandemic surveillance and reaction data to be able to determine resource needs.

71.   **The agriculture sector is affected by natural hazards that are expected to occur with increased frequency and severity due to climate change and requires special attention to enhance data availability.** In addition to hazard data, information on disaster damage and losses is also important to establish correlations between hazards and their consequences and develop risk models for agriculture.

72.   **The Hydrometeorological Service is in a good position to provide the data analytics required for the development of agriculture insurance.** The service has the data and technical capacity to provide sufficient data and agrometeorological advice for initial agriculture insurance, but more work is required. For example, the report "Agro-Climatic Resources of Batken Oblast of the Kyrgyz Republic" contains useful information for developing risk profiles for specific areas and crop/livestock types as well as for elementary insurance product design.[29] The service's website, however, is not informative, and it is difficult to find agriculture-related information that are easily available to the public.

> *Support the development of databases for agriculture risk management. Although weather and agriculture production data is available in the country, it is either in hard-copy format or needs redevelopment to be used for agriculture insurance . The database development activities should include data collection and storage, quality control, data processing and analysis, and data reporting.*

> *Increase the capacity of the Hydrometeorological Service to undertake the following:*

> - Conduct an analysis with the engagement of the insurance sector on the existing statistical data to identify gaps and quality issues as a basis for increasing the data usefulness for agriculture insurance provided by the service.
> - Develop digitized historical datasets (past 30 years) to be used for agriculture insurance and disaster risk management. These can also include factual data for more severe events with return period of more than 1-in-20 years.
> - Provide datasets to the agriculture insurance companies to be used for agriculture insurance, including data analysis, average annual loss estimation, and premium rate setting. This will be easier to implement if a subsidized agriculture insurance program is launched (para. 126), in which case the data can be provided to the agriculture insurance program administrator.

73.   **Insurance companies have not explored existing external sources of weather data, including weather data companies and suppliers of reanalyzed or satellite-derived weather datasets.**

> ***Insurers should obtain weather data from commercial weather data providers, which have historical and near-real-time weather data for the Kyrgyz Republic** (e.g., Meteoblue, Ubimet, IBM, AccuWeather, etc.)*

---

[29] Hydromet Kygyzstan, UNDP. Directory Agroclimatic Resources of Batken Oblast of Kyrgyz Republic (Russian version). http://upload.meteo.kg/attachment/83_93_eae0c7a3b5a80097e85d289cbc8c5670.pdf. (accessed 15 August 2022).

74.   **Agriculture insurance data is critical for the well-functioning of agriculture insurance, but it is not available.**

Require insurers to report agriculture insurance data separated by crop and livestock subtypes for both commercial and subsidized insurance program (if introduced). This could be done by individual companies or through the Insurance Association.

3.2 Government Policy

75.   **The government is aware of the need to support development of the insurance sector for it to efficiently support the economy and become a viable solution to finance disaster losses.** The Financial Market Supervision and Regulation Service of the Kyrgyz Republic (FSA) has formulated a proposal on the strategy to follow on 27 August 2020: "On approval of the Strategy for the Development of the Non-Bank Financial Market of the Kyrgyz Republic for 2020–2025." The strategy includes critical areas to be addressed such as the

- adoption of a new insurance law by the second quarter of 2022,[30]
- introduction of new solvency standards for insurers,
- creation and implementation of a new automated system at the FSA for collecting and processing reports from insurers,
- development and implementation of a software package for the identification and early warning of risks of deterioration in the financial condition of insurance companies,
- establishment of an insurance ombudsperson,
- creation of conditions that would encourage insurance companies to enter the pensions market, and
- participation of insurance companies in the compulsory health insurance system.

3.2.1 Households and Public Assets Disaster Risk Protection

76.   **Some 94 state-owned enterprises (SOEs) operate in the Kyrgyz Republic, and play a significant role in the local economy.** Many of them do not have disaster risk insurance. A combination of an underdeveloped insurance sector not offering adequate disaster risk products, including business interruption, and low demand leaves the large number of SOEs retaining disaster risk.

77.   **The existing compulsory insurance is weakly enforced.** The globally common types of mandatory insurance are present: workers compensation, civil liability insurance of carrier of dangerous goods, civil liability of organizations operating in hazardous production facilities, civil liability of the carrier to passengers—and the not very common but desirable disaster insurance of private homes. Motor third-party liability is being introduced on a staged basis. Enforcement of these types of compulsory insurance is poor (para. 81).

---

[30] The adoption of the new insurance law is delayed.

Disaster Home Insurance

78.   **In 2015, compulsory disaster insurance for private homes was signed into law.** The Law of the Kyrgyz Republic "On Compulsory Insurance of Accommodation Facilities Against Fire and Natural Disasters" (Compulsory Disaster Property Law) was approved on 31 July 2015, replacing the previous government mandate of providing grants and loans to people following disaster losses. Until 2015, the government had compensated people affected by disasters and accumulated significant liabilities. About $72 million was provided in loans from 2007 to 2014, with the number of outstanding loans steadily increasing over the years. In June 2015, the new disaster insurance law was approved. The Compulsory Disaster Property Law mandates household insurance against 18 types of hazards, including fire and natural hazards such as earthquakes, floods, mudslides, landslides, hail, etc.[31]

79.   **The government also established the State Insurance Organization to manage the program.** The annual premium for housing units in urban areas is set at Som1,200 ($15) and in the rural areas at Som600 ($7.55). The maximum limit of liability coverage in urban areas is set at Som1 million ($12,578) and in the rural regions at Som500,000 ($6,289). Based on government norms, socially vulnerable people receive government subsidies of 50% to 100% of the insurance premium. Note that organization retains all the risk without reinsurance.

80.   **According to State Insurance Organization data, over the last 5 years it has made payments on 530 insured events for a total amount of Som42 million ($4.953 million).** By the end of 2020, total insurance compensation paid over the years amounted to Som9,109.941 ($0.1 million) for the following causes:

- Wind, 65
- Fire, 34
- Mudflows, 18
- Snowfall, 4
- Hail, 1
- For other insured events, 19

  For 2 months in 2021 (January, and February), payments were made on 27 insured events amounting to Som2,934.987 ($36,400).[32]

81.   **Compliance with the mandatory disaster home insurance program has been extremely low.** As of November 2023, according to the Ministry of Emergency Situations, approximately 8% of all housing units had the mandatory coverage. According to the State Insurance Organization, extremely low compliance is primarily due to (i) lack of housing title documents; (ii) cultural factors; (iii) underdeveloped insurance sector and, thus, lack of confidence in insurance organizations; and (iv) lack of penalties for noncompliance. Box 5 outlines other bottlenecks in the home insurance program.

---

[31] That is, earthquake, flood (including caused by dam breaks), mudflow, avalanche, landfall, stone fall, landslide, increase of groundwater, strong wind, continuous rainfall, heavy rainfall and snowfall, snowstorm, and hail.

[32] State Insurance Company. https://gso.kg/en (accessed on 15 August 2022).

Box 5: Bottlenecks in the Home Insurance Program

Suboptimal claims process. This must be initiated by the household, with the household responsible for collecting all the necessary evidence, with State Insurance Organization (SIO) assistance. Evidence collection is quite cumbersome, e.g., testimonies from the Ministry of Emergency Situations and the local committee where the disaster took place, from the local meteorological station on weather conditions on the day of the event, and from the fire station in an event of a fire. The repayment requires an official loss assessment and the amount is determined following an SIO inspector's visit, and in accordance with Resolution 49 of February 2016 concurring to the percentage of the house area damaged, which structures are damaged (roof, etc.) and the type of damage incurred. The claim has to be settled within 30 days of all documents being submitted to the SIO. The amount depends on damage within the limits of the coverage.

Restricted underwriting. The policy will only be issued if a house fulfilled basic structural requirements, built with technical requirements. Houses located in areas classified as dangerous are excluded from the coverage.

Lack of knowledge on the use of the coverage. People are still in the process of learning the benefits of the coverage. For instance, the loss ratio remained low at around 10% between 2016 and 2019, with the exception of 2017, when it was 33%. Taking the 4-years activity into account, the loss ratio amounted to 15%.

Source: ADB. 2020. Preparing the Landslide Risk Management Project for the Government of the Kyrgyz Republic.

3.2.2 Diagnostic and Recommended Actions

82.   **The lack of disaster risk insurance of public assets, including the large number of SOEs, leaves the government exposed to possible severe losses due to extreme events such as major earthquakes.** The National Managing Company, a central holding company created in 2019 to manage all SOEs, has mandate to support especially poor-performing SOEs by facilitating more effective decision-making to attract management talent, additional resources, and investments in strategic SOE enterprises. Risk management capability is expected to be improved.

> *Using the risk layered approach, evaluate the use of insurance for critical public assets as a starting point toward securing insurance cover.* The National Managing Company is uniquely positioned to carry out assessment on disaster risk exposure of SOEs and acquire adequate DRF instruments in a centralized manner, including index and indemnity insurance, and business interruption.

83.   **The Compulsory Disaster Property Law and its implementation show deficiencies in achieving its objective for providing universal property insurance.** In 2018, the FSA undertook an analysis on the regulatory impact of the Compulsory Disaster Property Law and identified three options moving forward. Option 1 sees no changes made in the law, resulting in slow incremental growth in cover and the need for significant capitalization of the State Insurance Organization. Option 2 considers the opening of coverage to the private sector under the same conditions for all players. This would allow competition based on customer services and faster outreach growth; however, a critical question would be whether the existing insurers would be willing and able to offer cover in the area of low penetration. Under option 3,

coverage would be transferred to the government, thus, increasing government responsibility for household disaster protection as was the case before the Compulsory Disaster Property Law was established. This option would be contrary to supporting the need for an efficient disaster risk transfer product, and the needed creation of individual responsibility for DRF.

84.   **Option 1 is the most appropriate, but actions are required to implement it.** The Compulsory Disaster Property Law needs to be strengthened, as does State Insurance Organization's technical capacity to effectively implement it. For option 2, the insurance sector is currently in a nascent stage and would require further development before its participation in the Compulsory Disaster Property Law would be beneficial. Transfer of cover back to the government under option 3 would mean going back to the assistance and loans model that has already proven ineffective. Therefore, option 1 appears to be the best alternative subject to significant improvements.

Strengthen the Compulsory Disaster Property Law and enhance the State Insurance Organization's technical capacity through the following:

Solvency of the State Insurance Organization
- Assess the level of required capital according to the exposure assumed by the State Insurance Organization.
- Determine best mechanism to provide for required capitalization.
- Calculate the technical premium using an earthquake risk model when available.
- Buy reinsurance.

Improve State Insurance Organization processes to gain efficiency and wider acceptability
- Provide loss adjustment training.
- Develop a strategy to access sufficient loss adjusters if necessary.

Outreach of the Compulsory Disaster Property Law
- Improve enforcement of the law.
- Analyze impediments in the placement of the policy.
- Revise the sum insured on a regular basis considering building back better.
- Design a Compulsory Disaster Property Law awareness campaign.

Improve the Compulsory Disaster Property Law to increase acceptability
- Improve the claims payment process, including automatic claims payments (triggers could include magnitude of landslides, number of affected houses, number of lives lost).
- Design products with automatic claim payments and test them.

Enhance Compulsory Disaster Property Law benefits to target different sectors of the population
- Develop a product including retrofitting for houses in high disaster risk areas or with insufficient structural requirements.

- Consider a product where the construction firm should need to buy the Compulsory Disaster Property Law insurance for 5–10 years by paying a single premium.
- Design an additional plan for higher-end households.

Add optional benefits and price for them such as:
- Relocation in the form of a conditional money transfer: school attendance, medical visit, etc.
- Commuting costs.
- Income support to find a new job.
- Subsidies for basic food to offset increased cost of living for a transition period.
- Loss of income of the household due to infrastructure damage.

3.2.3 Epidemics and Pandemics Risk

Preparedness and Response

85.   **The Government of the Kyrgyz Republic has pandemic preparedness mechanisms in place, but the structures behind the policies are weak.** According to the Joint Evaluation of the International Health Regulation Core Capacities 2016 (WHO 2017). The Kyrgyz Republic scores high on areas such as health emergency plans and procedures, surveillance systems, and zoonotic diseases. However, solid implementation is hampered by lack of qualified staff and high staff turnover due to low salaries. Key areas for improvement are as follows:

- A whole-of-government approach in pandemic response, as responsibilities and structures are still operating in siloed mode and cross-sectoral links (such as security impacts, port-of-entry controls) are not addressed.
- The improvement of staffing norms and salaries, as these are limiting the country's ability to react efficiently (such as by deploying emergency staff and running reporting and surveillance chains).

86.   **The contingency funds within the budgets of the Ministry of Health and the Mandatory Health Insurance Fund proved to be insufficient for the COVID-19 pandemic.** Expenses in the pandemic were borne by the government and the international community. The Mandatory Health Insurance Fund received an additional Som2.1 billion in 2020 to cover additional expenses and employ more staff at facilities. The World Bank, ADB, and Islamic Development Bank provided international assistance. The Ministry of Emergency Situations was the main coordinating body in the government's management of the pandemic situation. While the Mandatory Health Insurance Fund received extra allocations from the government budget to cope with increased demand during the pandemic, COVID-19-related expenses were excluded in private health insurance policies.

87.   **In the wake of the pandemic, the Government of the Kyrgyz Republic reacted to the limitations during the pandemic.** In its National Development Plan (approved December 2021), the government addressed the following:

- Create sufficient stocks of commodities and personal protective equipment, alongside digitized and automated stock management systems.

- Create incentives for retaining staff at primary health care facilities to treat COVID-19 patients.
- Revise and improve relevant legislation considering lessons from the pandemic.
- Digitalize pandemic surveillance.
- Form of a single management center for pandemic emergencies.
- Introduce prevention and health promotion mechanisms, especially for vulnerable groups.

These measures are partly geared specifically to the COVID-19 pandemic and, thus, may not be sustainable (e.g., the staff incentives) as there is no budget increase for the health sector mentioned in the development plan.

The Health System Structure and Financing

88.   **The public health system provides a basic State Guaranteed Benefits Program to all citizens.** This comprises free emergency and primary, secondary, and tertiary care against co-payments in government facilities. Vulnerable groups such as children under 5, pensioners over 75, people with disabilities, as well as war veterans and many other similar groups, are exempt from co-payments. The exemptions are not poverty-specific (World Bank 2013 and OECD 2018). The State Guaranteed Benefits Program is financed through the Mandatory Health Insurance Fund under the Ministry of Health. Coverage for secondary and tertiary care is at 73% of the population (civil servants, formal employees, and other groups for whom the government pays the contributions). Primary health care coverage is 100%; however, some patients are unaware of their entitlements and/or prefer private providers for which they pay user fees. More than 70% of funds from the Mandatory Health Insurance Fund stem from the government budget, the remainder from member contributions, and the Social Fund (pension fund) (WHO 2018b).

89.   **All payments to public health facilities go through the Mandatory Health Insurance Fund.** In 2021, the Mandatory Health Insurance Fund had a regular budget of Som15.5 billion, and in 2022, Som19.9 billion. The Mandatory Health Insurance Fund contracts public facilities, and some private providers, for specialized treatments such as hemodialysis. Primary care outpatient services are paid on a per capita basis (capitation), and secondary and tertiary level inpatient services based on diagnosis-related case fees. As the payments from Mandatory Health Insurance Fund do not cover the facility cost, facilities raise official and informal co-payments (all co-payments being 39% of inpatient financing, the largest part informal co-payments) (World Bank 2019). The persistent underfunding of the Mandatory Health Insurance Fund compared with the actual treatment cost the facilities incur, and its high dependency on government payments, do not allow it to operate under actual insurance principles. Private health insurance cover is only marginal.

90.   **Health expenditure in 2019 was \$62 per capita,[33] the lowest in Central Asian states other than Tajikistan (Figure 10).** Of this, 51% was public, 46% was private out-of-pocket expenditure (outpatient drugs, co-payments), and 3% was private health insurance.

---

[33] World Bank National Health Accounts. Current Health Expenditure per Capita (current US\$)—Kyrgyz Republic | Data (worldbank.org) (accessed June 2022).

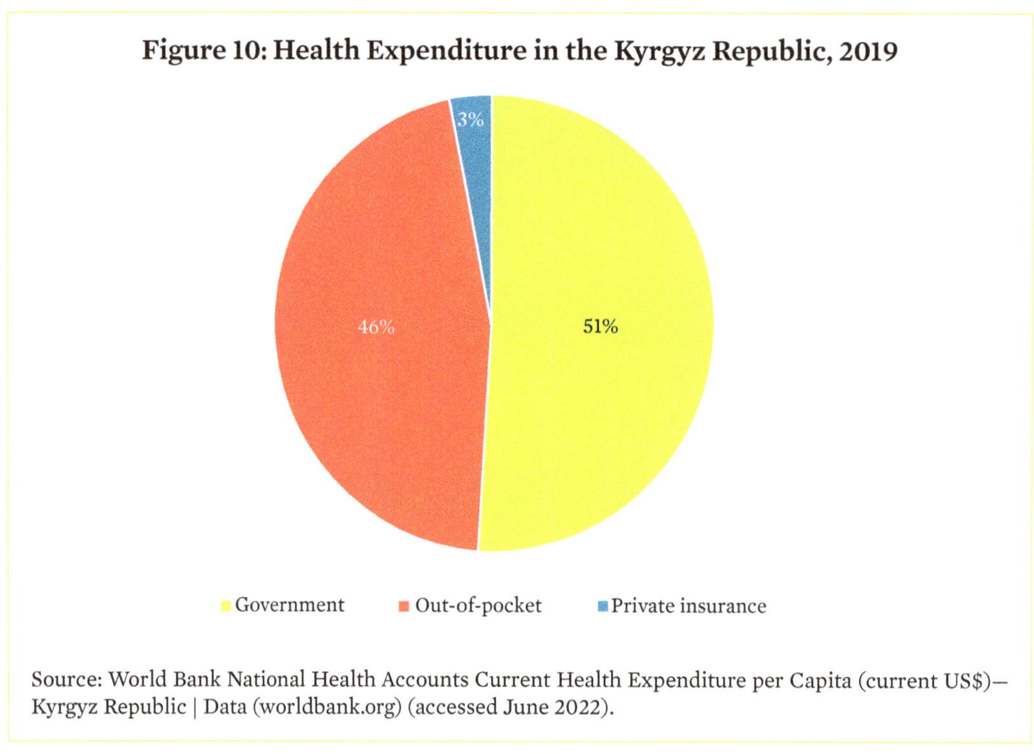

Figure 10: Health Expenditure in the Kyrgyz Republic, 2019

Source: World Bank National Health Accounts Current Health Expenditure per Capita (current US$)—Kyrgyz Republic | Data (worldbank.org) (accessed June 2022).

3.2.4 Diagnostic and Recommended Actions

91.   **Systems for pandemic preparedness are in place, but implementation is weak.**

Improve the integration of existing health emergency pillars.

92.   **Insufficient financing of basic health care creates vulnerabilities to manage pandemics and/or epidemics.** The main reason for the limited performance of the health emergency response systems lies with the underfunding of the health system, creating shortages in staff and commodities.

Work toward increased and sustainable health system financing, with a robust Mandatory Health Insurance Fund, adequate salaries, and sufficient means for commodity stocks.

93.   **The total cost of the Kyrgyz Republic's health response to COVID-19 is unclear, which makes understanding future epidemic and pandemic disaster-risk funding needs challenging.**

Develop a pandemics and/or epidemics financing plan based on a risk layered framework.

94.   **Pandemic and epidemic risk transfer instruments are not part of the sovereign DRF instruments.** The availability of such products is a challenge, due to the lack of geographical diversification of pandemic and epidemic risk (The Geneva Association 2021). Just by definition of epidemics and pandemics, diversification of the risk within a country or globally

is not possible, as seen for COVID-19, making geographic diversification not applicable for the management of this risk. Capital market investors, too, are likely to steer clear of pandemic risk transfer solutions, given their correlation with financial market impacts.

95.   **Time diversification of epidemic and pandemic risk is possible, due to the low frequency of severe epidemics and pandemics, but commercialization of such products is challenging.** Diversification in time requires the design of multiyear policies. Such policies themselves present important obstacles in their commercialization. Policies with a duration of more than a year are very seldomly written under the property line of business due to volatility in frequency and severity and because securing a commitment to pay for a premium over multiple years is demanding.

96.   **A complex payout design in line with the insurable interest principle is necessary.** In addition to the multiyear duration of the policies, the payout triggers need to match the financial demands generated by epidemics and pandemics in order to provide effective protection of the government budget. Thus, several payout triggers may be necessary in the presence of a declared epidemic or pandemic, relating to factors such as levels of bankruptcies, unemployment and hospital bed occupation rates. Designing such triggers that are objective, transparent, and not prone to fraud will need special dedication.

> ***Acquire sovereign pandemic and epidemic risk transfer instruments, which provide funds at the points of need if and when available.*** *Heavy reliance on development partner financing, although it was an important element of the recent COVID-19 response, may not be the optimum way of financing future events as such reliance may delay development projects.*

> ***At the same time, the availability of funds triggered by preventive health care needs will allow access to therapies in a timely way.***

3.2.5 Agriculture Risk Protection

Overview of Agriculture in the Kyrgyz Republic

97.   **Agriculture is responsible for "20% of total employment countrywide."**[34] "Despite its falling contribution to GDP, the agriculture sector remains important to community livelihoods and subsistence. About 60% of the population (about 6.5 million) is rural."[35]

98.   **The Kyrgyz Republic covers 199,951 square kilometers, with 5.8% forests, 4.4% water, 53.1% agriculture land, and 36% other lands.** Almost 90% of the territory is located 1,500 meters above sea level. "In 2018, total area under agriculture crops was 1.2 million hectares,"[36] with the largest crop areas located in Chui (34.5%), Issyk-Kul (15.1%), Osh (14.7%), and Jalal-Abad (12.8%) oblasts.

---

[31] Agriculture employment in 2018 is 20.3%, according to the National Statistical Committee of the Kyrgyz Republic. 2020. Specifics and Perspectives of Agricultural Sector Development in Kyrgyz Republic. https://stat.gov.kg/ru/news/tendencii-razvitiya-selskogo-hozyajstva-respubliki/.

[35] Food and Agriculture Organization of the United Nations. Country Fact Sheet on Food and Agriculture Policy Trends, February 2018. https://www.fao.org/agrifood-economics/publications/detail/en/c/1132131/.

[36] National Statistical Committee of the Kyrgyz Republic. 2020. *Specifics and Perspectives of Agricultural Sector Development in Kyrgyz Republic.*

99.   **High economic disparities between the rural areas of the north and south of the country exist—the north produces about 60% of the agriculture GDP, whereas the south produces less than 30% of the country's agriculture GDP (EU 2016).** The volume of gross output of agriculture, forestry, and fisheries in 2018 amounted to about Som205 billion ($2.5 billion) (IUJ and JICA 2020).[37] "The major agricultural regions in the country according to agricultural output value are Chui (25.4%), Osh (20.1%), and Jalal-Abad (19.9%) oblasts."[38] The combined agricultural output for these three regions is 65.4%.

100.   **Like many other developing countries, agricultural production in the Kyrgyz Republic is largely done by smallholder farmers with an average farm size of 3 hectares (World Bank 2018b).** According to the Kyrgyz Republic's National Statistical Committee, as of 1 January 2019, more than 440,000 economic entities operating in agriculture, forestry, and fisheries were registered. Of these, 333,000 or 75.6% were accounted for by farmer enterprises, of which 106,700 or 24.2% fell to individual businesspeople engaged in agriculture production. Osh oblast accounted for a significant proportion of agriculture business entities—120,800 or 27.5% of the total number of agriculture entities. Jalal-Abad oblast had 100,800 farms or 22.9%, and Chui oblast had 66,500 farms or 15.1% of the total number of agriculture producers in the country.[39]

101.   **In total, crop production accounted for 49.2% of total agriculture production, livestock products for 48.2%, forestry and fishery for 0.2%, and services for 2.4% (EU 2016).** The main crops produced in the Kyrgyz Republic in 2018 were cereals, potatoes, vegetables, cotton, tobacco, sunflower, and sugar beet.[40] Cereals were grown on about 50% of the arable land.

Agriculture Financing

102.   **The Government of the Kyrgyz Republic provides various types of support to the agriculture sector.** At time of the visit to the country, in 2022, there were six types of subsidies for agriculture and additional forms of tax relief:

- pest and crop management subsidies,
- financial support to seed producers,
- subsidies to breeding livestock farms,
- disease management subsidies,
- subsidized loans,
- subsidy payments to reduce water transport costs from the state water supply systems,
- land tax relief,
- income tax relief,
- profit tax relief,
- sales tax relief, and
- value-added tax relief.

---

[37] Exchange rate provided by XE.com.
[38] Footnote 36.
[39] Footnote 36.
[40] Footnote 36.

103.   **Annually, the government adopts a regulation that defines the volume of funds allocated from the state budget to support the agriculture sector.**[41] The most recent regulation was adopted in January 2022.[42] This document establishes the terms of financial support for the farmers. Government support is available to crop, livestock, and fish farmers, as well as to processing enterprises, including individual entrepreneurs. In 2018, the government allocated $2.35 billion to support investment in all sectors of the national economy. The agriculture sector was allocated 3.4% of the total budget (MOF 2018).

104.   **The subsidized loans are distributed through the commercial banks with the guarantees provided by the joint-stock company "Guarantee Fund."** Farmers and processors can get loans for a term of up to 60 months with an annual fixed interest rate of 6%. The difference between the interest rate offered to the farmers and processors and the market interest rate is compensated by the government to the commercial banks. Subsidized loans are available for crop, livestock, and fish production, the introduction of water-saving irrigation technologies, greenhouse operations, establishment and management of intensive orchards, organic production, purchase of livestock, purchase and storage of forage for livestock, etc. (MOF 2018).

105.   **Farmers can get access to commercial loans through banks and microfinance institutions.** Commercial loans have high interest rates (20% a year and higher), and short repayment periods, and so access to these financial services remains limited for small farmers, who often have modest financial management skills and unstable income (World Bank 2018b). Commercial banks and microfinance institutions use farm assets as collateral but do not consider crop or livestock insurance as additional security due to the underdeveloped agriculture insurance market. Finance providers commented that agriculture insurance can increase credit costs and make loan products too expensive for farmers and the rural population.[43]

Agriculture Sector Disaster Risk Protection

106.   **The Kyrgyz Republic is highly susceptible to disaster events such as avalanches, droughts, earthquakes, floods, and landslides, as noted.** Spring flooding occurs three to four times every year and affects most of the country's territory (CAREC Program 2022a). The agriculture sector is especially vulnerable to droughts, water shortages, and frosts. The Third National Communication by the Kyrgyz Republic highlights at least $14 million in average annual agricultural losses due to natural hazards during 1991–2011 (Kyrgyz Republic 2016).

---

[41] See the regulation on adoption of the project "Financing the Agricultural Sector – 9." 4 February 2021, #34 [in Russian]. http://cbd.minjust.gov.kg/act/view/ru-ru/158040; "Financing the Agricultural Sector – 8." 14 February 2020, #81. http://cbd.minjust.gov.kg/act/view/ru-ru/157700.

[42] See Regulation of the Cabinet of Ministers [Russian] http://cbd.minjust.gov.kg/act/view/ru-ru/218814.

[43] Feedback by the financial institutions received in during virtual project team mission in May 2022.

107.   **The agriculture sector faces several challenges.** These include socioeconomic vulnerability, lack of adequate infrastructure, lack of resources for farmers, land degradation, inadequate irrigation water supply, inefficient irrigation infrastructure, and food security. The focus of the National Sustainable Development Strategy of the Kyrgyz Republic, 2018–2040 for agriculture development is on overcoming limited abilities to produce sufficient agriculture commodities for food security and exports. This includes the lack of production facilities for traditional crops; and the introduction of systems for quality control of production, storage, and processing of agriculture products.

108.   **The government's agriculture policy (Food Security and Nutrition Program, 2019–2023) targets ensuring food security and an increase in nutritional self-sustainability.** In February 2021, the President issued a decree "on measures to develop the agro-industrial complex of the Kyrgyz Republic," which sets strategic objectives focusing on an increase in agriculture sector efficiency, pasture improvement, enhancement of farmers' access to new technologies, encouragement of public–private partnerships and establishment of logistics centers for agriculture commodities.

109.   **The Ministry of Emergency Situations is implementing a project together with the Food and Agriculture Organization of the United Nations (FAO) to enhance disaster risk reduction and preparedness in the agriculture sector.** The project started in 2019 to support climate change adaptation and ensure food security and better nutrition. The FAO will provide equipment (processors and computers) to establish a system for disaster data collection and maintenance of a database on different types of natural hazard in the country. The project also plans to analyze the impact of emergencies and natural hazards on the agriculture sector.

110.   **Recognizing the importance of climate and weather risk management in the agriculture sector, the government has proposed legislative initiatives to develop agriculture insurance but most have yet to gain traction.**

- The government drafted a law on crop insurance in 2009.[44] This law sets the terms of insurance with government support including a 50% subsidy to reduce the premium cost to agriculture producers. The law was not accepted by farmers and insurance companies and was never implemented.
- In a decree "On the measures to develop the agro-industrial complex of the Kyrgyz Republic" adopted on 8 February 2021 (#25), the President suggested that the government must implement measures to introduce agriculture insurance (article 1, para. 5).
- In 2021, a new draft law on agriculture insurance was developed by the Ministry of Agriculture. The ministry suggested to make a decision on the potential model of agriculture insurance with the government support in the country. This draft law introduces the classification of agriculture insurance types, terms of insurance with government support, and the concept of a standard insurance product. This draft law is still at discussion stage and it is not known when it will be sent to the Parliament for adoption.
- In 2011, the Ministry of Agriculture developed a draft law on livestock insurance but it was not adopted.

---

[44] The law on specifics of insurance in crop production (Закон "Об особенностях страхования в растениеводстве"), #31. 26 January 2009.

3.2.6 Diagnostic and Recommendations

111.   **Increasing financial protection for farmers is critical.** As indicated in para 97, around 20% of the population are employed in the agriculture sector. The sector is highly exposed to disaster risk, and especially to hydro-meteorological events, which are expected to become more frequent and severe due to climate change. As an important and critical point, agriculture insurance needs to be developed to ensure sustainability of the agriculture sector. Notwithstanding the usefulness of agriculture insurance, this instrument is far from a panacea for farmers to manage risk. A holistic approach is needed.[45]

112.   **The country lacks a disaster risk management framework for disasters affecting agriculture.** The increasing frequency and severity of disasters affecting agriculture, such as floods, droughts, and landslides, requires all aspects of disaster risk management to be implemented simultaneously. The management of such risks effectively is not possible without a clear DRF mechanism. The management of high frequency, low severity risks like non-extreme floods and droughts requires dynamic ex ante DRF instruments including insurance as well as ex post DRF mechanisms. The Kyrgyz Republic needs to formulate a disaster risk management policy for agriculture that encapsulates the unique aspects of the country's agriculture reality.

Develop the DRF framework for agriculture based on the risk layered approach.

3.3 Credibility of the Private Sector Offering Risk Transfer Solutions

3.3.1 Insurance Regulation and Supervision

113.   **Insurance regulation and supervision is carried out by the Financial Market Supervision and Regulation Service of the Kyrgyz Republic (FSA).** The FSA evolved from the State Service for Regulation and Supervision of the Financial Market under the Ministry of Finance and Economy of the Kyrgyz Republic. According to Chapter 7 of Resolution No 659 of 31 December 2018, "On Questions of the Activities of the State Service of Regulation and Supervision of the Financial Market under the Government of the Kyrgyz Republic," the FSA is an independent agency funded by the state budget. The agency is split into three divisions, one of which deals with licensing, another with auditing companies, and the third with proposed legislation. A senior specialist heads each division. The FSA has been a member of the International Association of Insurance Supervisors (IAIS) since 2006.

114.   **The primary legislation on insurance activity are the Civil Code of the Kyrgyz Republic and the Law of the Kyrgyz Republic "On Organization of Insurance in the Kyrgyz Republic."** The Civil Code covers the overview of the insurance market, licensing

---

[45] "Agricultural crop insurance is a restricted instrument in that it only addresses production and yield losses because of weather and natural risks, providing limited coverage for the growing crop from the time of sowing or crop emergency through to completion of harvest. It does not however usually address downstream sources of risks including post-harvest storage losses, or market price risk. It (insurance) can only address part of the losses resulting from some perils and is not a substitute for good on-farm risk-management techniques, sound production and farm management practices, early weather forecasts and investment in technology" (M. Tuladhar 2015).

provision, liquidation, and operational aspects of insurance businesses. The law establishes the basic principles of state regulation of insurance activities.

115.   **The solvency requirements are primitive and need to be developed for supervision to be effective.** Articles 17 and 18 of Law No 96 "On the Organization of Insurance in the Kyrgyz Republic" dated 1998, require insurers to comply with the solvency requirements as developed by the FSA. Currently, insurers are required to hold assets in excess of their liabilities at least totaling the minimum capital requirements and liability for an individual risk in an insurance contract cannot exceed 20% of an insurer's own funds.

116.   **Minimum authorized capital is set out in Regulation No. 292 "On Minimum Capital Requirements of Insurance (Reinsurance) Companies and Insurance (Reinsurance) Broker" dated 7 June 2016:**

- For an insurance organization that carries out activities on voluntary types of insurance and/or reinsurance, with the minimum capital should be exception of life-saving life insurance, at least Som30 million ($397,000).
- For an insurance organization that carries out voluntary and mandatory insurance and reinsurance activities, including life insurance, the minimum capital should be at least Som150 million ($1.98 million).
- For an insurance organization that carries out activities solely for reinsurance, it should be at least Som300 million ($3.97 million).
- For insurance (reinsurance) broker, it should be at least Som1 million ($13,000).

3.3.2 Diagnostic and Recommended Actions

117.   **The FSA's significant amount of work to regulate, supervise, and develop the insurance sector in a sound manner requires important capacity building and significant resources.**

Assess the current and future resources and expertise needed by the FSA to carry out effective supervision of the insurance sector and to provide guidance and support for the sector to develop, and implement the findings.

118.   **Prudential regulation does not observe the IAIS principles.** Currently, the solvency requirements do not address the inherent risk taken by the insurers.

Assess the regulation and supervision of the insurance sector against IAIS principles and implement the findings.

3.3.3 The Insurance and Reinsurance Sector

Insurance

119.   **The insurance sector is one of the smallest in the world, with $17 million premium in 2020 of which 68% was property insurance and less than $2,000 life premium.** Total assets were less than $60 million or 0.6% of GDP as of 2019. Insurance penetration was just 0.23% in 2018. Notwithstanding the low premium volume, 17 insurance organizations operate

in the market, with the strong dominance of Ingosstrakh,[46] which held 45% of market share as of 2021. The market only reached two-digit growth in 2019 and was then severely impacted by the COVID-19 pandemic, resulting in near no growth in 2020 (Table 4).

Table 4: Insurance Premium, 2016–2020
(Som million)

Premium	2016	2017	2018	2019	2020	2020 ($ million)
Nonlife	829	877	940	1153	1181	15.30
Personal Accident & Health	91	129	158	180	154	1.99
Total	920	1,006	1,098	1,333	1,335	17.29
Growth	4.81%	8.55%	8.38%	17.63%	0.15%	
Assets	2,730	4,395	3,993	4,859	. . .	57.21

. . . = not available.
Source: AXCO. 2022. Non-life Insurance Market Reports Kyrgyzstan.

Reinsurance

120.   **Reinsurance has been provided by foreign companies since the 2018 closing of the two local reinsurers.** The market exiting of the two reinsurers, Strakhovoi Reserv and Favorit, was replaced by international reinsurers active in the market. Notwithstanding the elimination of the 5% minimum retention requirement, leading to several risks now being 100% reinsured, the reinsurance premium decreased from 61% in 2016 to 50% (2019) of the direct premium (Som675 million in 2019, last data available) (Table 5).

Table 5: Reinsurance Premium, 2016–2019
(Som million)

	2016	2017	2018	2019
Reinsurance	564.97	533.55	505.03	673.97
Retention ratio	39%	47%	54%	49%

Source: AXCO. 2022. Non-life Insurance Market Reports Kyrgyzstan.

121.   **Regulation requires insurers to reinsure in excess of 20% of any one risk.** This is a prudential measure given that the solvency regime does not reflect the risks assumed by the insurers.

---

[46] Ingosstrakh" Insurance Joint-Stock Company was established in 1996 as a joint venture with "Ingosstrakh" Insurance Company (Moscow), as well as a member of "INGO" International Insurance Group. At the end of 2021, Ingosstrakh assets amounted to Som890 million with Som334 million equity.

Pools

122.   **There are no insurance pools operating in the Kyrgyz Republic.**

3.3.4 Diagnostic and Recommendations

123.   **The size of the insurance sector limits its importance in disaster risk financing protection.** According to the CAREC Risk Profile Report (CAREC Program 2022a), the average annual loss to flood in the Kyrgyz Republic is assessed at $73.3 million, while the average annual loss to an earthquake is assessed at $72.4 million. UNESCAP estimates the average annual loss to drought at $186.5 million.[47] The average annual loss assumptions suggest that the average annual loss associated with the major hazards (flood, earthquake, and drought) to be funded is equal to around $332.2 million. The expected average annual loss is thus 5.5 times higher than total assets ($60 million in 2019) of the insurance sector or 24 times higher than the total annual premium ($17 million in 2020). (Note that there might be years with much higher losses than the average annual loss that will require either reinsurance or capital inflows.)

Develop a strategy to grow the insurance sector and implement it.

3.3.5 Private Health Insurance Sector

124.   **Private health insurance exists only marginally in the Kyrgyz Republic.** There are policies for outpatient and inpatient treatments available that cover additional costs such as co-payments, drugs, etc., or treatments that are not part of the State Guaranteed Benefits Program. However, few insurance providers offer exclusively corporate schemes and they mainly serve as staff incentives or salary component. Uptake is further hampered by the limited administrative readiness of health facilities (e.g., to produce an invoices of co-payments paid that could be processed by an insurer). Demand for private individual health insurance is also minimal, due to the low-income status of the country.

3.3.6 Agriculture Insurance

125.   **Agriculture insurance is nascent, with an insignificant premium volume of a few thousand US dollars.** There is no special insurance class or subclass for agriculture insurance as can be found in other countries. This is because the volumes of agriculture insurance are unknown due to insufficient public data although some sources suggest that the total annual agriculture insurance premium is about $15,000. Insurance companies are interested in offering agriculture insurance but they lack skills and knowledge. There is a lack of qualified agriculture underwriters, portfolio managers, and loss adjusters.[48]

3.3.7 Diagnostic and Recommendations

126.   **The development of agriculture insurance as a globally proven DRF tool is critical to support sustainable farming.** Since the Kyrgyz Republic is almost at the starting point as

---

[47] UNESCAP. Kyrgyz Republic: Risk Profile. https://www.unescap.org/sites/default/files/Kyrgyzstan%20 Disaster%20Risk%20Profile.pdf.

[48] This feedback was provided by insurance companies during virtual mission meetings in May 2022.

far as agriculture insurance is concerned, it can learn from global experience and design an effective National Agriculture Insurance Program, spearheaded by the government.

Develop agriculture insurance including crop, livestock, and fishery. The following actions are recommended:

Adopt the law on agriculture insurance currently in discussion to introduce a public-private partnership framework for the agriculture insurance program. *The success of the government-supported program will be subject to financial availability and the introduction of institutional capacity to administer an agriculture insurance program. The current draft law can stimulate the introduction of the agriculture insurance program but it requires legislative adoption and continuous support from the government side.*

Subsidize agriculture insurance. *The international practice provides that the allocation of subsidies for agriculture insurance helps to establish an agriculture insurance program quicker and achieve more sustainable results in the long run.*

Establish an agriculture insurance pool to develop agriculture insurance. *The pool could be jointly funded by the insurance industry, the Government of the Kyrgyz Republic, and development partners.[49] This option appears particularly interesting for the Kyrgyz Republic given that agriculture insurance is hardly available in the market. The pool could start piloting various product and process innovations. Over the long term, the pool could graduate into a full-fledged crop and livestock insurance company. Thus, an agriculture insurance pool could provide underwriting capacity for increasing penetration of agriculture insurance, including by providing a modern product offering, centralized data gathering on agriculture risk, and strong negotiation power for reinsurance protection.[50]*

Develop technical competency to support the development of agriculture insurance. *This should include knowledgeable staff within relevant government agencies to administer the state-supported agriculture insurance program. The insurance companies will need to train agriculture insurance underwriters, actuaries, and loss adjusters and create a regional network to offer agriculture insurance products in rural regions. This work can be implemented jointly by insurance companies, government agencies, and development partners.*

---

[49] Risk transfer solutions in agriculture needs specialized exclusive providers to be effective. Agriculture insurance is a highly specialized business and may require substantial investments in technology, actuarial, and risk management expertise with regard to agriculture. Further, the inherent covariance of agriculture risk in the form of perils affecting all or almost all insured in an area (like price and weather risk) limits the ability of risk sharing with the few farmers not affected by the losses. Therefore, several countries have implemented risk transfer solutions in agriculture through risk pools that increase the outreach of products and geographic area.

[50] The international reinsurance companies can provide more favorable terms of reinsurance for agriculture programs with the development potential and premium volumes over $500,000. This level of agriculture insurance premium is achievable even if only 1% of agriculture output would be insured. (This assumption is based on the annual value of agriculture production of $2.5 billion in 2018 and the average premium rate of 3% [$2.5 billion x 1%] x 3% = $750,000 of premium).

Take advantage of new technologies to develop agriculture insurance and enhanced risk management (Figures 11, 12, and 13). *These technologies include reanalyzed weather datasets (to supplement the existing weather data), which are available from various weather data companies; drones and satellite remote sensing for agriculture asset management and disaster events monitoring; and geographic information system (GIS) technologies for managing the agriculture insurance and subsidy programs. Information technologies can be considered for agriculture subsidy applications and management, portfolio management, and disaster response. Such systems have already been introduced in other developing countries (e.g., Indonesia, Kazakhstan, the Philippines, etc.) and it is possible to replicate such solutions in the Kyrgyz Republic.*

Figure 11: Satellite Optical Image of Irrigated Maize Fields

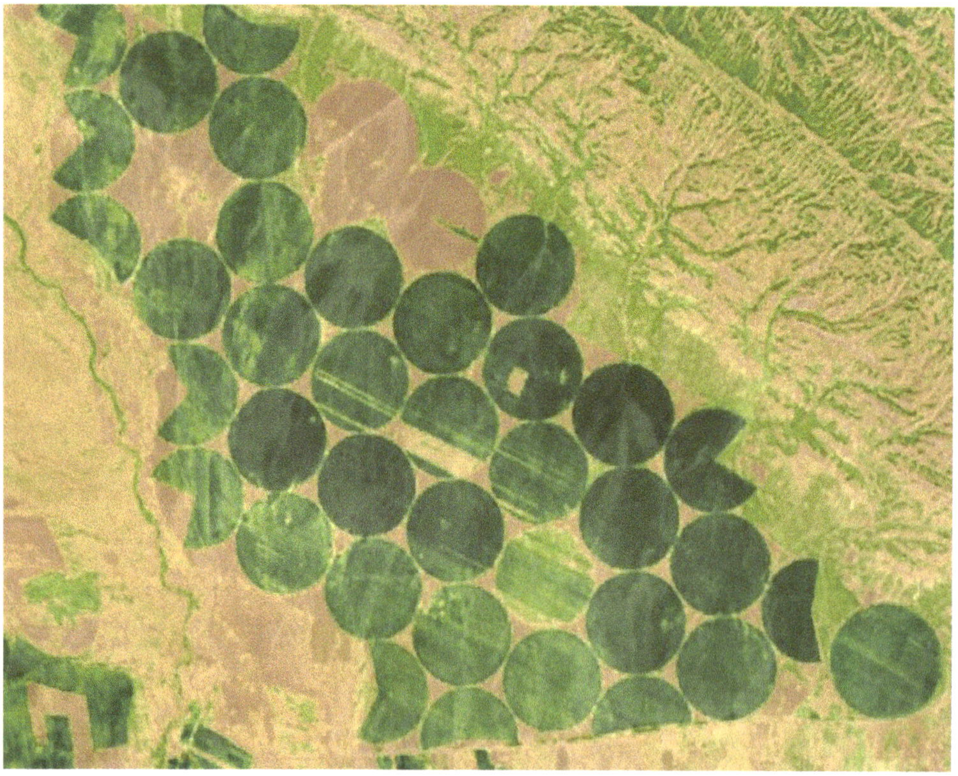

Source: Agroinsurance International LLC.

**Figure 12: Photo of Maize Fields Taken by Drone Showing Problem
Areas of the Fields**

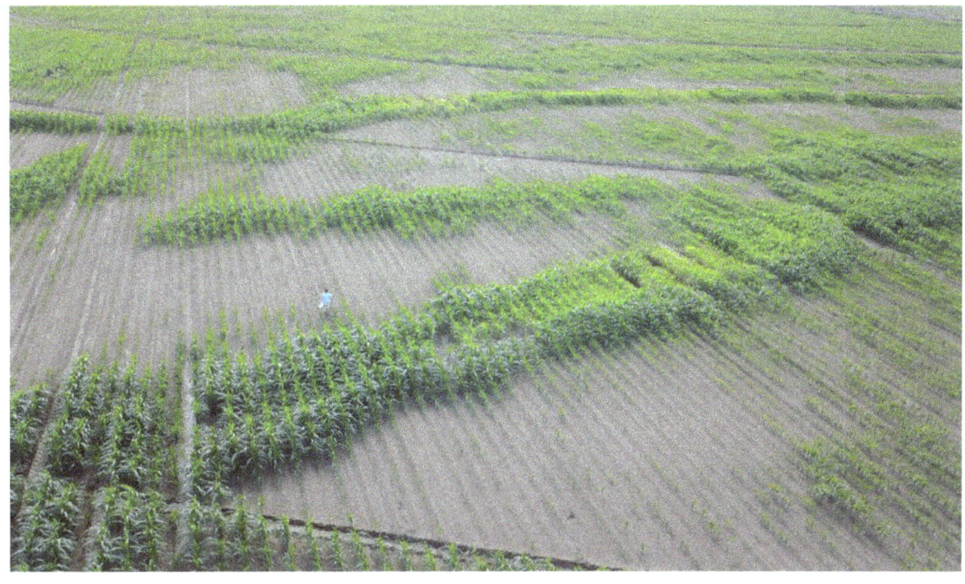

Source: Agroinsurance International LLC.

Figure 13: Satellite Image Showing Problem Zones in a Vineyard

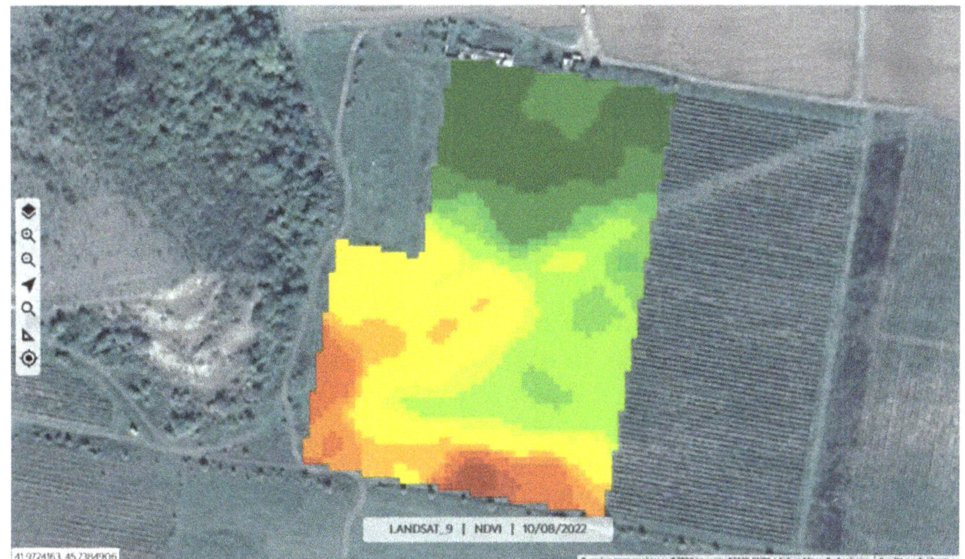

green = good crop condition, red and orange = problem areas.
Note: Normalized Difference Vegetation Index (NDVI).
Source: Agroinsurance International LLC, EarthDaily Agro.

3.4 Product Availability and Affordability

127.   **The insurance sector offers a range of products but, other than the Compulsory Disaster Property Law, no disaster insurance protection is available.** Besides the compulsory insurance, voluntary products include

- health insurance,
- property insurance,
- motor insurance,
- aviation risk insurance,
- construction and installation insurance,
- cargo insurance,
- liability insurance of road carriers,
- employee accident insurance,
- liability insurance of warehouse owners and terminal operators,
- professional liability insurance, and
- general liability insurance.

128.   **Insurance availability for higher value risk depends on reinsurance accessibility.** The insurers' limited capacity requires the use of reinsurance when accepting high value risks or specialty products. Thus, insurers follow the reinsurers' price, which sometimes is economically prohibitive for the population. Large multinational risks are 100% fronted. The reinsurers' underwriting guidelines imposed on the market following international practices exclude risks that cannot be diversified, such as pandemics, war, nuclear events, etc. Special exceptions are possible, but at a high cost and most commonly found in multinational insurance programs.

3.4.1 Catastrophic Risk Insurance Products

129.   **Beside the Compulsory Disaster Property Law, no disaster risk products are present in the market.**

3.4.2 Diagnostic and Recommendations

130.   **While the use of pools is common practice in several countries to deal with insurance market failures in areas such as agriculture, energy, aviation, or disaster risk, the Kyrgyz Republic does not use this type of instrument.**

> *Consider setting up effective risk pools to support the development of agriculture insurance and disaster risk products (para. 126). The pool will increase the available capacity of the market, provide stronger negotiation power when purchasing reinsurance, create a center of technical expertise, and centralize historical claims data.*

3.4.3 Health Insurance Products

131.   **There are no local private individual health insurance products available.** Insurers offer corporate insurance schemes. Other than that, there are only international health insurance products available, at international premium rates.

3.4.4 Diagnostic and Recommended Actions

132.   **The insurance sector is currently too small to provide adequate health insurance products for individuals.**

> *Attract international health insurance providers to offer and develop individual health plans including for pandemics and/or epidemics.* *The incentives could include special licensing for offshore operations.*

3.4.5 Agriculture Insurance Products

133.   **The existing agriculture insurance in the country is minimal.** Agriculture crop insurance is provided by two companies,[51] and three companies provide livestock insurance. The crop insurance premiums are in the range of 0.5% to 2.0% of the insured amount while livestock premium ranges from 3% to 5% of the sum insured. Notwithstanding the existing premium subsidy from the government of 50% for agriculture producers, the uptake is very low and the few developed agriculture insurance product prototypes have not been introduced mainly due to lack of technical capacity, data availability and the high cost of the risk.[52] Furthermore, many insurance applications are rejected due to the lack of an independent harvest-weighing system and the low number of customers. As a result, farmers are exposed to disasters and expect the government to provide support in the event of losses. Disaster impact is especially severe for small subsistence farmers. No evidence of fisheries insurance was found.

3.4.6 Diagnostic and Recommended Actions

134.   **Development of agriculture insurance products faces serious challenges requiring several actions to be taken.**

> - *Develop a suite of standard insurance products for the agriculture insurance program.* *Standard insurance products respond to established expectations, create faster understanding of the product, and help to make public awareness campaigns more effective. Standardized products allow private insurance companies to introduce the required procedures and processes quicker and more efficiently with fewer resources required for research and development. The suite of products should be designed to meet the needs of various farmers' groups. The products may include indemnity (named-peril, multi-peril), index, parametric, and hybrid solutions.*[53]

---

[51] The Jubilee Kyrgyzstan Insurance Company and the University of Central Asia, with the German insurer Hannover Re and the Humboldt University of Berlin, are piloting a weather index-based agriculture insurance scheme as part of a regional project funded by the Government of Germany and implemented from 2017 to 2020: KlimALEZ. Increasing Climate Resilience in Central Asia - Sustainable Rural Development through the Introduction of Innovative Agricultural Insurance Product.

[52] For instance, an insurance company considered a weather index insurance product for wheat several years ago. The product was designed by one of the leading reinsurance companies. The product concept was discussed with farmers but received unfavorable feedback. This initiative was put on hold and no index insurance was offered at the market.

[53] Index insurance can be suitable at the meso and macro levels to establish the overall disaster mitigation framework. The area-yield index can be a pragmatic insurance solution for field crop growers on condition the yield assessment for loss adjustment purposes can be introduced effectively. The named-peril or multi-peril crop insurance can be a suitable option for commercial farmers growing strategic field and high-value crops but this will require the development of insurance infrastructure to support the traditional insurance products offering.

- *Introduce the products gradually, starting with products for the larger crop and livestock types (based on area planted, livestock population number), especially for those with food security importance.*
- *Develop standard underwriting, especially standard loss adjustment procedures for agriculture insurance.* Loss adjustment is often a particular source of problems and disputes if farmers do not understand the loss adjustment procedures or the insurance companies do not use standard procedures.

3.4.7 Business Interruption Insurance

135.   **Business interruption or loss of income insurance is not offered in the Kyrgyz Republic as a stand-alone product.** The standard product is linked to fire or property insurance and the payout under the business interruption policy requires physical damage of the property. Pandemic-related business interruption or loss of income is, thus, not covered. The public awareness of the benefits of business interruption is also low and the underwriting of business interruption or loss of income requires transparency in the income of the insured, which is a challenge in most developing countries.

136.   **Significant uninsured business revenue losses have drawn attention to business interruption insurance globally.** The COVID-19 measures in the form of lockdowns, limits on the size of gatherings, travel restrictions, etc., have led to approximately $1.7 trillion in revenue losses as estimated by the OECD (OECD 2021). As noted, the pandemic led to the contraction of output by 8.4% in 2020, a substantial loss of jobs, with 80% reduction in tourism. Without risk transfer instruments, and to protect massive business closures and liquidations as well as exploding unemployment rates, governments globally responded with significant financial support programs. The need for business interruption or loss of income insurance has drawn public attention.

3.4.8 Diagnostic and Recommended Actions

137.   **Lack of pandemic risk diversification and low demand for business interruption insurance needs to be overcome for a viable risk transfer solution.** Having highlighted the difficulties to providing coverage for the financial impact of pandemics, this does not rule out the provision of small-scale, selected private market coverage by limiting the degree of risk transfer and the number of businesses covered. Such availability of the product would benefit the country.

> *Initially, the government rather than individual companies should consider acquiring multiyear coverage for business interruption that includes pandemics and/or epidemics (paras. 94–96).*

3.4.9 Travel Insurance

138.   **Standard travel insurance policies exclude epidemics and pandemics risk.** One of the main reasons for this exclusion is the fact that when epidemics and pandemics are declared, they become a known event, contradicting the central principle of insurance that it should cover events that have not occurred or do not have a 100% probability of occurrence for the duration of the policy. However, for COVID-19, the requirement in several countries to have travel insurance policy that covers COVID-19, related costs has led insurance companies

to design such a product. This has been possible due to the strict conditions for travel, like full vaccination, negative testing, and quarantine.

3.4.10   Diagnostic and Recommended Actions

139.   **Due to greater awareness of epidemics and pandemics risk, future travel insurance policies will have to include undeclared epidemics and pandemics in their coverage.** This will only be possible at an affordable price if conditions are in place that mitigate the risk of infections due to travel-related pandemic exposure, i.e. full vaccination, negative testing etc.

Require future travel insurance policies to include undeclared epidemics and pandemics in their coverage.

3.4.11   Capital Markets Supporting Disaster Risk Financing

140.   **The Kyrgyz Stock Exchange (KSE) has been in operation since 1995 but remains small.** The KSE was founded in 1994 in the form of a non-state, nonprofit organization, supported in its establishment by the State Supervision Agency 28 companies are listed issuing stock and bonds, mainly banks and subnational companies, as well as two microfinance companies. There are 33 investment instruments (as of July 2022) traded by 19 market participants including security brokers, investment companies, finance companies, and stock brokers. Total domestic market capitalization amounted to $407.16 million (as of 2022).

141.   **The KSE trade volume is growing, albeit with an erratic pattern that remains small.** Total annual trade volume reached Som14 billion ($180 million) in 2022 based on the second quarter 2022 trade volume (Figure 14 and Table 6). Bank lending and international development partner financing remain the primary mechanisms by which businesses in the Kyrgyz Republic seek to fund expansion projects.

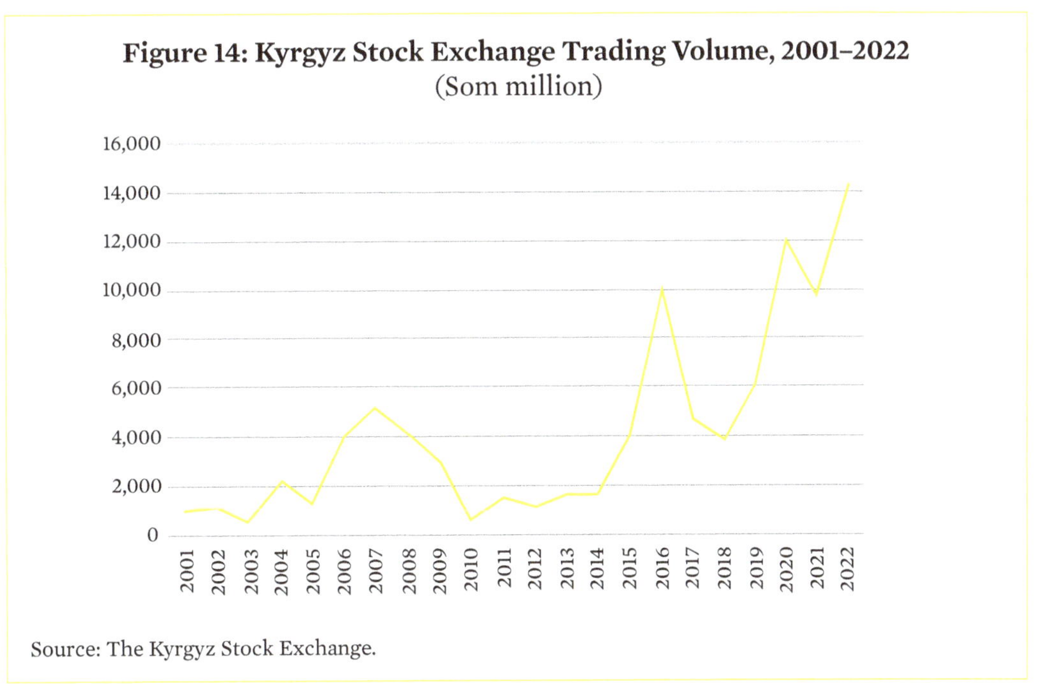

Figure 14: Kyrgyz Stock Exchange Trading Volume, 2001–2022
(Som million)

Source: The Kyrgyz Stock Exchange.

Table 6: CSX Trading Statistics, 2001–2022
(Som1,000)

Year	Total Trade Volume	Number of Securities	Number of Transactions	Trades on the Primary Market	Trades on the Secondary Market	Trades of Listed Securities	Trades of Non-listed Securities
2001	941,304.70	85,228,814.00	6,599.00	537,928.09	403,376.69	144,202.20	797,102.40
2002	1,129,340.99	47,029,516.00	3,167.00	324,513.20	804,827.81	426,059.60	703,281.59
2003	511,892.91	48,818,669.00	1,877.00	149,288.40	362,604.31	102,731.60	409,161.60
2004	2,209,320.33	44,899,366.00	2,305.00	1,233,184.80	976,135.61	301,327.60	1,907,992.74
2005	1,245,809.51	51,008,715.00	1,745.00	630,200.61	615,608.89	562,266.88	683,542.31
2006	3,916,302.16	139,430,925.00	2,284.00	1,180,491.02	2,735,810.96	840,749.31	3,075,552.86
2007	5,188,567.71	364,048,384.00	4,092.00	1,502,203.41	3,686,364.11	988,350.30	4,200,217.33
2008	4,183,776.05	390,967,002.00	3,408.00	924,146.30	3,259,629.52	595,892.51	3,587,883.34
2009	2,951,189.54	428,968,255.00	926.00	1,528,100.00	1,423,089.51	842,806.70	2,108,383.01
2010	459,712.79	900,602,256.00	693.00	69,483.50	390,229.39	97,478.30	362,234.71
2011	1,511,016.69	451,032,719.00	1,678.00	690,313.30	820,703.40	860,942.97	650,074.00
2012	1,169,382.48	393,642,682.00	2,185.00	330,769.80	838,612.59	398,648.89	770,733.70
2013	1,648,139.00	91,734,881.00	3,325.00	777,149.40	870,989.50	663,260.40	984,878.81
2014	1,634,300.88	330,134,204.00	3,516.00	1,129,510.12	504,790.90	39,284.90	1,241,457.92
2015	4,007,882.71	157,878,477.00	1,948.00	2,716,038.76	1,291,844.09	2,926,380.01	1,081,502.50
2016	9,969,352.48	749,649,656.00	1,821.00	8,026,602.99	1,942,749.57	1,630,893.70	8,338,458.90
2017	4,643,749.04	146,307,573.00	1,526.00	3,524,288.38	1,119,460.71	2,649,105.27	1,994,643.78
2018	3,801,826.08	338,332,735.00	2,953.00	3,036,564.47	765,261.69	2,458,097.28	1,343,728.79
2019	6,073,948.15	166,173,818.00	2,726.00	5,845,127.14	228,820.80	4,425,915.38	1,648,032.62
2020	11,830,783.06	280,365,163.00	1,413.00	11,452,638.18	378,144.90	4,724,058.72	7,106,723.98
2021	9,738,175.27	136,077,666.00	2,032.00	9,207,338.71	530,836.69	3,729,824.07	6,008,351.51
2022*	14,290,030.77	309,706,798.00	2,299.20	13,053,449.86	1,236,581.60	10,249,646.59	4,040,384.352
Total:	93,055,803.00	6,052,038,274.00	54,518.20	67,869,330.44	25,186,473.24	40,011,481.18	53,044,322.75
15 Aug 2022	8,931,269.23	193,566,749.00	1,437.00	8,158,406.16	772,863.50	6,406,029.12	2,525,240.22

Source: Kyrgyz Stock Exchange.

3.4.12   Diagnostic and Recommended Actions

142.   **The KSE has limited capacity to develop and trade catastrophe bonds or other insurance-linked securities.** With current trading of 33 domestic investment instruments in the form of stock or bonds, limited trade volume and Moody's downgrading of the Kyrgyz Republic's sovereign credit rating to B3 in January 2022, domestic capital market solutions to support DRF with capital market products are not expected in the short or medium term.

Explore and take advantage of regional initiative to develop catastrophe bonds and other insurance-linked securities to enhance the DRF instruments, especially for extreme but infrequent events, like a major earthquake (para. 52).

143.   **The government has expressed its desire to develop a green economy to contribute to sustainable economic growth.** This presents a unique opportunity to consider the development of special bonds, particularly given the government's revised, more ambitious Nationally Determined Contributions as presented at the 26th United Nations Climate Change Conference of the Parties (COP26) in November 2021. These include a goal to reduce greenhouse gas emissions by 17% by 2025 under the business-as-usual scenario and by 37% subject to international support (financial assistance) (Box 6).

Box 6: Climate Change Mitigation and Adaptation Efforts

The effort, as unveiled at the 26th United Nations Climate Change Conference of the Parties (COP26) in November 2021, will focus on the three sectors that produce the most greenhouse gas emissions: energy, agriculture, and forestry and other types of land use.

The Kyrgyz Republic has abundant water resources that the government plans to develop sustainably to increase the share of hydropower in its energy mix. Other plans include increased carbon flow from populated areas toward forests by creating new forest plantations and expanding the areas with perennial forest, and areas cultivated under organic land farming.

The Kyrgyz Republic joined the Global Methane Pledge in 2021. Although the government has committed to reaching net-zero carbon emissions by 2050, it has not announced or debuted any policy measures to achieve this goal. The mission is unaware of any public procurement policies that include environmental and green growth considerations.

Most regulatory incentives to encourage clean energy development and climate-friendly business practices involve tax breaks and credits.

Source: U.S. Department of State.2022. *Investment Climate Statements: Kyrgyz Republic.* https://www.state.gov/reports/2022-investment-climate-statements/kyrgyz-republic/.

3.5 Social Protection Policy

3.5.1 Government Protection Plans for the Low-Income Population

144.   **Social protection in the Kyrgyz Republic is wide-ranging as social protection is seen as a basic right of all citizens.** Social protection programs in the Kyrgyz Republic include both contributory and noncontributory elements under the main three pillars: social insurance, social assistance, and labor market policies—the social insurance segment being the most significant pillar. The government also provides public access to widespread health care services. The government spends more public resources on social protection than any other area (OECD 2018). As Table 7 shows, public expenditure on social protection amounted to over Som11 billion ($138.5 million) in fiscal year 2020 and Som12.35 billion ($155.3 million) in fiscal year 2021, while Som15.55 billion ($195.6 million) were approved for fiscal year 2022. Expenditure on social protection accounted for nearly 7% of total public spending in fiscal year 2020 and 4% in fiscal year 2021, while approved budget for social protection for fiscal year 2022 accounted for nearly 5% of the total approved Republic Budget.

Table 7: Public Expenditure on Social Protection

2020	2021	2022
Total Expenditures	Total Expenditures	Approved Budget
Som11,008,488,001	Som12,346,470,000	Som15,553,364,000
$138,471,044	$155,301,509	$195,639,799

Source: Government of the Kyrgyz Republic, Ministry of Finance.

145.   **As of 2022, the only explicit social protection mechanism in place to support people affected by disasters is the mandatory disaster home insurance program.** This is detailed under subsection 3.5.1. Under this program, the government offers 50% to 100% subsidies of the insurance premium to socially vulnerable people. Compliance with the program has been slow—as of November 2022, according to the Ministry of Emergency Situations, only 8% of all housing units were covered by the insurance.

146.   **The government provides limited cash payments to people affected by disasters, primarily through the President, Prime Minister, and Parliament funds.**[54] During disasters, local authorities in coordination with Ministry of Emergency Situations prepare lists of people affected by disasters and submit them to the relevant Parliament committees for approval. In 2021, for instance, following major floods, 200 families received Som150,000 from the President's Fund and Som50,000 from that of the Prime Minister—about $2,500 per family in total. The process to identify affected people is cumbersome, as it requires certification by multiple local and central authorities. Additionally, in response to COVID-19, the government's measures included emergency health spending, a food security program, temporary tax deferrals and subsidized loans to small and medium-sized enterprises, liquidity support to banks, deferrals of loan payments, and the temporary relaxation of capital and loan provisioning norms (IMF 2021). In 2020, for instance, the Ministry of Health and Social Development (MHSD) "provided one-off food assistance to 523,880 newly poor and vulnerable beneficiaries through 1227 hotline" (WFP 2021). Development partners also provide humanitarian assistance to people affected by disasters (subsection 2.3.3.).

147.   **The government is evaluating the entire social protection system.** Currently, the Kyrgyz Republic does not have a national social protection development strategy, while the Social Protection Development Programme of the Kyrgyz Republic for 2015–2017 has not been renewed. However, the 2021 Action Plan for the National Development Programme to 2026, adopted through a Presidential decree, includes a planned "evaluation of social protection system of the population for compliance with international norms and standards" (Task No. 698 under the Inclusive Growth section) to identify minimum social protection levels and provide the basis for the development of a national social protection development strategy. Preparation for the evaluation is underway with technical assistance from the development partners involved in social protection in the Kyrgyz Republic—in particular, the World Bank, the International Labour Organization (ILO), the World Food Programme (WFP), and the United Nations Children's Fund (UNICEF).

---

[54] Resources allocated to these funds, or the amounts allowed to be spent through them, are not disclosed.

3.5.2 Diagnostic and Recommended Actions

148.   **An integrated national social protection strategy is critical to avoid fragmentation and enhance poverty-targeting effectiveness, but has not been implemented.**

> ***Develop and implement an integrated national social protection strategy.*** *The strategy should streamline the current social schemes, making them more poverty-sensitive and relying on integrated structures (databases, payout mechanisms, and beneficiary selection).*

149.   **The social protection might be crowding out the private sector.** The allocated public funding is an indication of the wide social engagement of the government, however, as pointed out by a UNICEF assessment, it faces a number of challenges, which include the following:

- Social protection programs are too narrow in scope, with targeting errors and implementation difficulties.
- Social assistance suffers from fragmentation, low coverage, and low transfer values—thus, does little to tackle poverty.
- Social care services have been underdeveloped with prevailing residential care. Outreach and effectiveness of case management need to be improved.
- Social service workforce needs systemic reform and modernization (UNICEF 2022).

> ***Consider engaging the private sector to supplement and replace selected areas of the social protection like the pensions and certain workers' benefits to increase the premium volume and, hence, resources of the insurance sector.***

3.6 Unlicensed Competition

150.   **Insurance activity is a regulated activity under the law "On organization of insurance in the Kyrgyz Republic."** While the regulator has not reported any unlicensed insurance activity, the notable absence of life insurance offered locally indicates that the upper sector of the population may be consuming this type of insurance abroad.

3.6.1 Diagnostic and Recommended Actions

151.   **Unlicensed activity is possibly addressing the unmet need for life insurance given that the local life business in the country is virtually nonexistent.**

> ***Monitor offshore life business to limit any negative impact on the development of the life insurance sector.***

4 Conclusions

4.1 Rating Summary and Recommended Main Actions

152. **The ideal enabling environment for disaster risk financing (DRF) coincides with the achievable scenario for the Kyrgyz Republic.** For this reason, the gap analysis of the current scenario has been carried out against the ideal scenario. Based on the insights gained by applying the W&W diagnostic tool, no differences between the ideal scenario and the realistic or achievable scenario were found. Responses from stakeholders regarding the realistic scenario were more by way of providing additional solutions for achieving the ideal environment scenario, rather than describing limitations that would hinder realization of the ideal. The figure presenting the ratings, thus, shows only the current situation versus the ideal enabling environment (Figure 15).

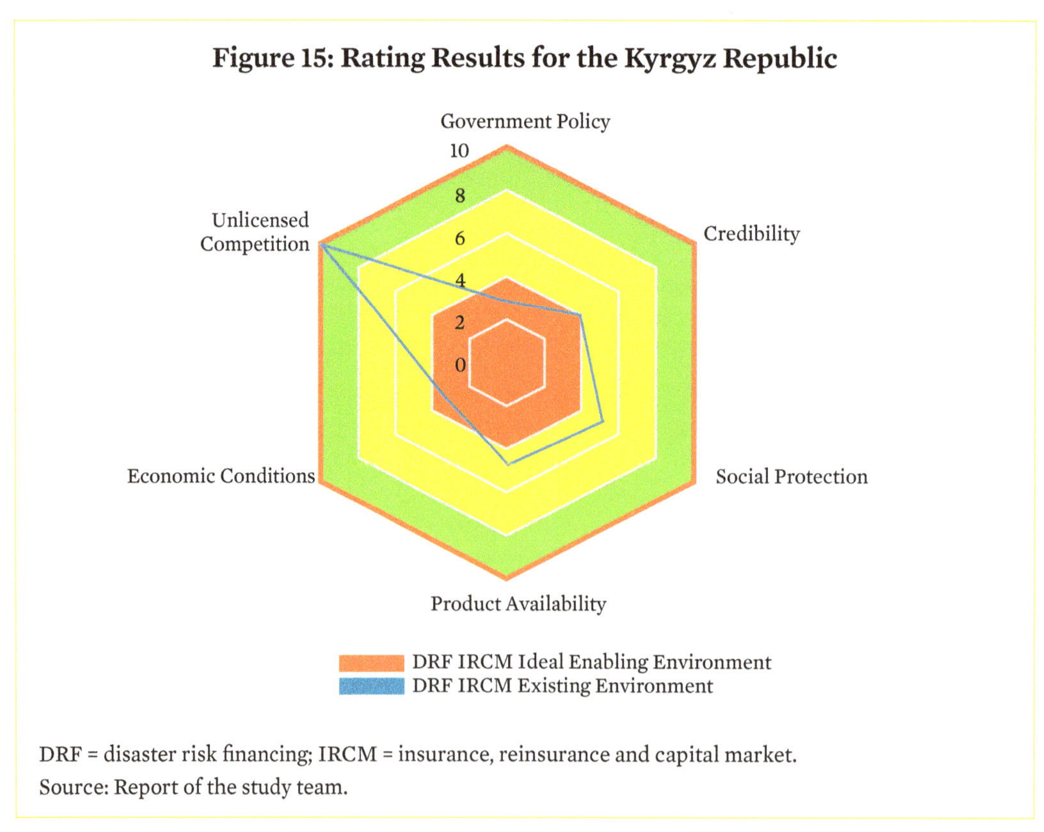

Figure 15: Rating Results for the Kyrgyz Republic

DRF = disaster risk financing; IRCM = insurance, reinsurance and capital market.
Source: Report of the study team.

4.1.1   Economic and Other Preconditions

- **The rating is in the red zone, implying urgent need for action (section 3.1).**

Main gaps identified:

- Insufficient insurance professionals is limiting the ability of insurers to develop disaster risk insurance products.
- Investments in weather monitoring infrastructure are insufficient.
- Substantial agritech progress in other countries has led to smarter insurance products to protect livelihood and income of farmers.
- The availability and access to disaster risk models provides the basis for a robust DRF strategy and the pricing of insurance premiums.
- The existing health information landscape and pandemic surveillance data systems are still fragmented and partly manually operated.
- The agriculture sector is affected by natural hazards that are expected to occur with increased frequency and severity due to climate change, and this requires special attention with respect to enhanced data availability.
- Insurance companies have not explored existing external sources of weather data, including weather data companies and suppliers of reanalyzed or satellite-derived weather datasets.
- Insurance companies have not explored existing external sources of weather data, including weather data companies and suppliers of reanalyzed or satellite-derived weather datasets.
- Agriculture insurance data is critical for the well-functioning of agriculture insurance, but it is not available.

Main recommended actions to close the gaps:

- Establish a strategy to develop insurance professionals.
- Increase investments in weather monitoring infrastructure to support DRF mechanisms.
- Develop agritech to reduce risk to a level where insurance becomes sustainable and affordable.
- Collect necessary data from the relevant governmental ministries on disaster events affecting the country.
- Develop an open source disaster risk model covering all major hazards, including pandemics and/or epidemics faced by the country.
- Develop and implement a health information systems integration strategy.
- Support the development of databases for agriculture risk management and increase the capacity of the Hydrometeorological Service.
- Insurers should obtain weather data from commercial weather data providers, which have historical and near-real-time weather data for the Kyrgyz Republic.
- Require insurers to report agriculture insurance data separated by crop and livestock subtypes for both commercial and subsidized insurance program (if introduced).

4.1.2 Government Policy

- **The rating is in the red zone, implying urgent need for action (subsections 2 and 3.2).**

- Existing budget allocations are insufficient to enable the government to retain fiscal shocks arising from annual disaster events.
- The financing of infrequent but severe disaster events need attention.
- There is limited information related to fiscal risks arising from disasters.
- The lack of disaster risk insurance of public assets, including the large number of state-owned enterprises, leaves the government exposed to possible severe losses.
- The Compulsory Disaster Property Law and its implementation show deficiencies in achieving its objective for providing universal property insurance.
- Systems for pandemic preparedness are in place, but the implementation is weak.
- Insufficient financing of basic health care create vulnerabilities to manage pandemics and/or epidemics.
- The total cost of the country's health response to COVID-19 is unclear, which makes understanding future epidemic and pandemic disaster-risk funding needs challenging.
- Pandemic and epidemic risk transfer instruments are not part of the sovereign DRF instruments.
- Increasing the financial protection for farmers is critical.

Main recommended actions to close the gaps:

- Explore options for securing a contingent disaster financing facility.
- Acquire risk transfer solutions for the extreme but infrequent disaster events.
- Enhance the collection of information and related analysis regarding fiscal risks arising from disaster.
- Using the risk layered approach, evaluate the use of insurance for critical public assets as a starting point toward securing insurance cover.
- Increase the resilience of the State Insurance Organization.
- Improved the State Insurance Organization's processes to increase efficiency and acceptability.
- Enforce the law to improve its outreach.
- Enhance the Compulsory Disaster Property Law benefits to target different sectors of the population.
- Improve the integration of existing health emergency pillars.
- Work toward an increased and sustainable health system financing with a robust Mandatory Health Insurance Fund, adequate salaries, and sufficient means for commodity stocks.
- Develop a pandemics and/or epidemics financing plan based on the risk layered framework.
- Acquire, at government level, pandemic and epidemic risk transfer instruments that provide funds at the points of need when available and if economically viable.
- Develop the DRF framework for agriculture based on the risk layered approach.

4.1.3   Credibility in the Insurance Sector and the Capital Markets

- **The rating is in the red/yellow border zone, implying urgent need for action (subsection 3.3).**

Main gaps identified:

- The significant amount of work of the Financial Market Supervision and Regulation Service of the Kyrgyz Republic (FSA) to regulate, supervise, and develop the insurance sector in a sound manner requires important capacity building and significant resources.
- Prudential regulation does not observe the principles of the International Association of Insurance Supervisors (IAIS).
- The size of the insurance sector limits its importance in disaster risk financial protection.
- The development of agriculture insurance as a globally proven DRF tool is critical to support sustainable farming.

Main recommended actions to close the gaps:

- Assess the current and future resources and expertise needed for an effective supervision.
- Carry out an assessment of the regulation and supervision against the IAIS principles and implement the findings.
- Develop a strategy to grow the insurance sector and implement it.
- Develop agriculture insurance including crop, livestock, and fishery.

4.1.4   Products

- **The rating is in the yellow zone, implying need for action (subsection 3.4).**

Main gaps identified:

- While the use of pools is common practice in several countries to deal with insurance market failures in areas like agriculture, energy, aviation, or disasters, the Kyrgyz Republic does not use this type of instrument.
- The insurance sector is currently too small to provide adequate health insurance products to individuals. Significant business revenue losses have remained uninsured.
- Travel insurance excludes pandemics.
- The Kyrgyz Stock Exchange has limited capacity to develop and trade catastrophe bonds or other insurance-linked securities.
- The government has expressed its desire to develop a green economy to contribute to sustainable economic growth.

Main recommended actions to close the gaps:

- Consider to set up effective risk pools to support the development of agriculture insurance and disaster risks products.

- Attract international health insurance providers to offer and develop individual health plans.
- Develop a suite of standard insurance products for the agriculture insurance program.
- Introduce gradually the products, starting from the larger crop and livestock types.
- Develop standard underwriting and, especially, standard loss adjustment procedures for agriculture insurance.
- Consider multiyear business interruption insurance for the government.
- Require future travel insurance policies to include undeclared epidemics and pandemics in their coverage.
- Explore and take advantage of regional initiative to develop catastrophe bonds and other insurance-linked securities to enhance the DRF instruments, especially for extreme but infrequent events, like a major earthquake.

4.1.5 Social Protection

- **The rating is in the yellow zone, implying need for action (subsection 3.5).**

Main gaps identified:

- An integrated national social protection strategy is critical to avoid fragmentation and enhance poverty-targeting effectiveness but has not been implemented.
- The social protection might be crowding out the private sector.

Main recommended actions to close the gaps:

- Develop and implement an integrated national social protection strategy.
- Consider engaging the private sector to supplement and replace selected areas of the social protection like the pensions and certain workers' benefits.

4.1.6 Unlicensed Competition

- **The rating is in the green zone, implying no action is needed (subsection 3.6).**

Main gaps identified:

- Unlicensed activity is probably replacing the absence of life business in the country.

Main recommended actions to close the gaps:

- Monitor offshore life business as part of a development strategy of the life sector.

References

Alliance for Hydromet Development and World Bank Group. 2021. Country Hydromet Diagnostics, Kyrgyz Republic, 2021 Peer Review. https://alliancehydromet.org/wp-content/uploads/2021/07/Kyrgyz-report.pdf.

Asian Development Bank (ADB). 2013. *Investing in Resilience: Ensuring a Disaster-Resistant Future.*

——. 2020. *TA-9726 KGZ: Preparing the Landslide Risk Management Project for the Government of the Kyrgyz Republic.*

——. 2021. *COVID-19 and the Finance Sector in Asia and the Pacific.* https://www.adb.org/sites/default/files/institutional-document/761946/covid-19-finance-sector-asia-pacific-guidance-note.pdf.

——. Forthcoming. Toolkit for Insurance, Reinsurance and Capital Market Solutions for Disaster Risk Financing, Assessing the Enabling Environment for Disaster and Pandemic Risk Financing– A Country Diagnostics Toolkit (Revised version).

ADB and the World Bank. 2017. *Assessing Financial Protection against Disasters: A Guidance Note on Conducting a Disaster Risk Finance Diagnostic.*

Bank for International Settlements (BIS). 2020. *Annual Report Economic Report 2020.* https://www.bis.org/publ/arpdf/ar2020e1.pdf.

Burunciuc, Lilia. 2020. Natural Disaster Cost Central Asia $10 Billion a Year—Are We Doing Enough to Prevent Them? *World Bank Blogs.* 5 November. https://blogs.worldbank.org/europeandcentralasia/natural-disasters-cost-central-asia-10-billion-year-are-we-doing-enough.

CAREC Program. 2022a. *Country Risk Profile, Kyrgyz Republic.* CAREC Secretariat, ADB, Manila. https://www.carecprogram.org/uploads/CAREC-Risk-Profiles_Kyrgyz-Republic.pdf.

CAREC Program. 2022b. *Narrowing the Disaster Risk Protection Gap in Central Asia.* CAREC Secretariat, ADB, Manila. https://www.adb.org/sites/default/files/publication/821771/disaster-risk-protection-gap-central-asia.pdf.

European Union (EU). 2016. Action Document for the Integrated Rural Development Program (IRD) in Kyrgyz Republic.

Free, Matthew, Katherine Coates, and Yannis Fourniadis. 2018. Seismic Risk in the Kyrgyz Republic, Central Asia, Conference Paper. *Semantic Scholar.*

The Geneva Association. 2021. *Public-Private Solutions to Pandemic Risk: Opportunities, Challenges and Trade-Offs.* https://www.genevaassociation.org/sites/default/files/research-topics-document-type/pdf_public/pandemic_solutions-report_final.pdf.

GFZ Helmholtz Centre Potsdam. 2020. Early Warning System for Dams at Risk. Press release. 17 December. https://www.gfz-potsdam.de/en/press/news/details/early-warning-system-for-dams-at-risk.

Holzhacker, H. and D. Skakova. 2019. Kyrgyz Republic Diagnostic. European Bank for Reconstruction and Development.

International Budget Partnership. 2021. *Managing COVID Funds: The Accountability Gap.* https://internationalbudget.org/covid/wp-content/uploads/2021/05/Report_English-2.pdf.

International Energy Agency (IEA). 2020. Kyrgystan Energy Profile, Country Report.

International Monetary Fund (IMF). 2021. Kyrgyz Republic: 2021 Article IV Consultation-Press release and Staff Report.

International University of Japan and Japan International Cooperation Agency (JICA). 2020. The Possibility of "Six Sector Industrialization" in Kyrgyzstan Agricultural Products. https://www.academia.edu/43568449/The_Possibility_of_Six_Sector_Industrialization_in_Kyrgyzstan_Agricultural_Products.

Kompas, T., V.H. Pham, and T.N. Che. 2018. The Effects of Climate Change on GDP by Country and the Global Economic Gains from Complying with the Paris Climate Accord (2018). https://agupubs.onlinelibrary.wiley.com/doi/full/10.1029/2018EF000922.

Kyrgyz Republic. 2016. Third National Communication to the United Nations Framework Convention on Climate Change.

Kull, D., T. Jukusheva, and N. H. Naqvi. 2022. Learning from the Kyrgyz Republic's Efforts to Strengthen its Weather Forecasting Service. *World Bank Blog.* 19 April. https://blogs.worldbank.org/europeandcentralasia/learning-kyrgyz-republics-efforts-strengthen-its-weather-forecasting-service.

Laatikainen, T., L. Inglin, I. Chonmurunov, B. Stambekov, A. Altymycheva, and J. L. Farrington. 2022. National Electronic Primary Health Care Database in Monitoring Performance of Primary Care in Kyrgyzstan. *Primary Health Care and Research Development.* 23 (e6). National Library of Medicine. https://www.ncbi.nlm.nih.gov/pmc/articles/PMC8822322/.

Lillis, J. 2022. Central Asia to Suffer Remittances from Russia Nosedive. *Euroasianet.org.* 11 March. https://eurasianet.org/central-asia-to-suffer-as-remittances-from-russia-nosedive.

Ministry of Finance (MOF). 2018. Civil Budget for 2018 in the Kyrgyz Republic [in Russian]. http://www.minfin.kg/.

Organisation for Economic Co-operation and Development (OECD). 2018. *Social Protection System Review of Kyrgyzstan.* https://www.oecd.org/countries/kyrgyzstan/Social_Protection_System_Review_Kyrgyzstan.pdf.

———. 2019. Sustainable Infrastructure for Low-Carbon Development in Central Asia and the Caucasus: Hotspot Analysis and Needs Assessment. Chapter 5. Investment in Sustainable Infrastructure in the Kyrgyz Republic. https://www.oecd-ilibrary.org/sites/8b30e9f8-en/index.html?itemId=/content/component/8b30e9f8-en.

——. 2021. Responding to the COVID-19 and Pandemic Protection Gap in Insurance. 16 March. https://www.oecd.org/coronavirus/policy-responses/responding-to-the-covid-19-and-pandemic-protection-gap-in-insurance-35e74736/.

Parolai, S., T. Boxberger, M. Pilz, and K. M. Fleming. 2017. Assessing Earthquake Early Warning Using Sparse Networks in Developing Countries: Case Study of the Kyrgyz Republic. *Frontiers in Earth Science*. 5 (74). https://www.researchgate.net/publication/319933310_Assessing_Earthquake_Early_Warning_Using_Sparse_Networks_in_Developing_Countries_Case_Study_of_the_Kyrgyz_Republic. https://www.preventionweb.net/collections/covid-19-and-natural-hazards.

Public Expenditure and Financial Accountability (PEFA). 2021. *Kyrgyz Republic Performance Assessment Report.* https://www.pefa.org/sites/pefa/files/2021–10/KG-Aug21-PFMPR-Public%20with%20PEFA%20Check.pdf.

Reliefweb. 2008. Kyrgyz Quake Raises Questions over Shoddy Buildings. Press release. 17 October. https://reliefweb.int/report/kyrgyzstan/kyrgyz-quake-raises-questions-over-shoddy-buildings.

Tuladhar, M. 2015. Need for Sustainable Service Model to Promote Agriculture Insurance. New Business Age. 2 April 2015.

United Nations Children's Fund (UNICEF). *Kyrgyzstan. Disaster Risk Reduction.* https://www.unicef.org/kyrgyzstan/disaster-risk-reduction.

United Nations Development Programme (UNDP). 2022. National Disaster Risk Reduction Strategy Action Plan 2023–2026 Was Discussed. https://www.undp.org/kyrgyzstan/press-releases/national-disaster-risk-reduction-strategy-action-plan-2023–2026-was-discussed#:~:text=The%20concept%20of%20comprehensive%20protection%20of%20the%20population%20and%20territory,January%2029%2C%202018%20%E2%84%96%2058.

United Nations Economic and Social Commission for Asia and the Pacific (UNESCAP). 2021. Infrastructure Financing in Kyrgyzstan. https://www.unescap.org/sites/default/d8files/event-documents/Infrastructure%20Financing%20in%20Kyrgyzstan.pdf.

United Nations Framework Convention on Climate Change (UNFCC). 2016. Kyrgyz Republic Third National Communication to the UNFCCC. https://unfccc.int/sites/default/files/resource/NC3_Kyrgyzstan_English_24Jan2017_0.pdf

——. 2022. Submission to the UN Special Rapporteur on Extreme Poverty and Human Rights.

University of Notre Dame. 2020. *Notre Dame Global Adaptation Initiative.* https://gain.nd.edu/our-work/country-index/.

U.S. Department of State. 2022. *Investment Climate Statements: Kyrgyz Republic.* https://www.state.gov/reports/2022-investment-climate-statements/kyrgyz-republic/.

Wehrhahn, R. 2010. Insurance Underutilization in Emerging Economies: Causes and Barriers. In C. Kempler, M. Flamée, C. Yang, and P. Windels (eds.). *The Global Perspectives on Insurance Today: A Look at National Interest versus Globalization.* Palgrave Macmillan.

World Bank. 2013. *Toward Universal Coverage in Health: The Case of the State Guaranteed Benefit Package of the Kyrgyz Republic.* https://documents1.worldbank.org/curated/en/685631468278090377/pdf/750060NWP0Box30l0Coverage0in0Health.pdf.

———. 2017. *Kyrgyz Republic, Measure Seismic Risk.* https://documents1.worldbank.org/curated/en/911711517034006882/pdf/Kyrgyz-Republic-Measuring-seismic-risk.pdf.

———. 2018a. *Boosting Financial Resilience to Natural Disasters in Central Asia.* News feature. 31 July. https://www.worldbank.org/en/news/feature/2018/07/31/boosting-financial-resilience-to-natural-disasters-in-central-asia.

———. 2018b. Climate-Smart Agriculture for the Kyrgyz Republic. https://climateknowledgeportal.worldbank.org/sites/default/files/2019–06/CSA%20_Profile_The%20Kyrgyz%20Republic.pdf.

———. 2019. *Toward a More Pro-Poor and Explicit Health Benefit Package in the Kyrgyz Republic.* Washington D.C. https://openknowledge.worldbank.org/server/api/core/bitstreams/52d3c3d6–2911–52c9-af2f-e5cfa0b70780/content.

———. 2020. Public Expenditure Review. Creating fiscal space for inclusive growth. https://openknowledge.worldbank.org/bitstream/handle/10986/35789/Kyrgyz-Republic-Public-Expenditure-Review-Creating-Fiscal-Space-for-Inclusive-Growth.pdf?sequence=1&isAllowed=y.

———. 2022. *Sustaining Small Business through the Pandemic in Kyrgyz Republic.* Feature Story. 6 May 2022. https://www.worldbank.org/en/news/feature/2022/05/06/sustaining-small-business-through-the-pandemic-in-kyrgyz-republic#:~:text=The%20country's%20poverty%20rate%20is,opportunities%2C%20have%20been%20hit%20hard

World Bank and ADB. 2021. *Climate Risk Country Profile for Kyrgyz Republic.* https://www.adb.org/sites/default/files/publication/706596/climate-risk-country-profile-kyrgyz-republic.pdf.

World Food Programme (WFP). 2021. *Poverty, Food Security and Nutrition Analysis in the Context of COVID-19 and the Role of Social Protection in the Kyrgyz Republic.* https://docs.wfp.org/api/documents/WFP-0000133148/download/?_ga=2.197369199.1350292497.1680514232–343521517.1680514232.

World Health Organization (WHO). 2017. Joint External Evaluation of IHR Core Capacities of the Kyrgyz Republic (Mission report). https://extranet.who.int/sph/sites/default/files/documentlibrary/document/JEE%20Report%20Kyrgyzstan%202016.pdf

———. 2018a. *Quality of Care Review in Kyrgyzstan, Working Document.* https://www.euro.who.int/__data/assets/pdf_file/0004/383890/kgz-qoc-eng.pdf.

———. 2018b. *Can People Afford to Pay for Health Care?* https://www.euro.who.int/__data/assets/pdf_file/0007/381589/kyrgyzstan-fp-eng.pdf.

www.ingramcontent.com/pod-product-compliance
Lightning Source LLC
Chambersburg PA
CBHW041836110726
48006CB00020B/2640